# AND IN HEALTH

# AND IN HEALTH

## A Guide for Couples Facing Cancer Together

Dan Shapiro, PhD

TRUMPETER
Boston & London  2013

Trumpeter Books
An imprint of Shambhala Publications, Inc.
Horticultural Hall
300 Massachusetts Avenue
Boston, Massachusetts 02115
www.shambhala.com

9 8 7 6 5 4 3 2 1

First Edition
Printed in the United States of America

♾This edition is printed on acid-free paper that meets the American
National Standards Institute z39.48 Standard.
♻This book is printed on 30% postconsumer recycled paper. For more
information please visit www.shambhala.com.

Distributed in the United States by Random House, Inc.,
and in Canada by Random House of Canada Ltd

Designed by Daniel Urban-Brown

LIBRARY OF CONGRESS CATALOGING-IN-PUBLICATION DATA

Shapiro, Dan, 1966–
And in health: a guide for couples facing cancer together /
Dan Shapiro, PhD.—First edition.
Pages   cm
ISBN 978-1-61180-017-3 (pbk.)
1. Cancer—Patients—Family relationships. 2. Couples.
3. Caregivers. I. Title.
RC262.S458 2013
616.99'4–dc23
2012043419

For Terry, who held my hand when the storms came.
And came again.

He is the cheese to my macaroni.

—Diablo Cody, *Juno: The Shooting Script*

# Contents

# Acknowledgments

I am grateful to the many couples and individuals who shared their experiences and generously allowed me to tape and quote them. Notably, every person I spoke with contributed a piece of wisdom. Over the years I've also learned a great deal from courageous patients who came to me for couples counseling. Their insights formed the backbone of the book. I thank Alma Jeanne Brandt and Dee Bailey, who transcribed all of the interviews. Dee Bailey developed an organizational scheme and while doing so noticed a few themes I'd neglected, and those became chapters. Dr. Kimberly Myers read the entire manuscript and provided line-by-line suggestions and, as always, optimistic, practical, and insightful feedback. I am also grateful to my agent, Rebecca Friedman, who gave early input, and to my hard-working editor, Jennifer Urban-Brown, who helped sculpt the manuscript. Finally, I am grateful to my family, who are, by now, accustomed to being exposed in my writing and still live with me despite this.

# AND IN HEALTH

# Introduction

Cancer will take you places you never thought you'd go.

—NANCY N.

She had a double mastectomy eight days ago. The surgery recovery has been painful, but now, for the first time in weeks, she feels frisky. And on a deeper level, she wants to feel sexy and attractive after spending the past week in hospital gowns tethered to IV poles.

*Maybe these painkillers are loosening me up a little too.* No matter, she's going to have some fun. She carefully puts on the black underwear he likes with the cut that runs high on her thigh and wears a sweatshirt so that she can still move despite the tight bandages wrapped around her chest over the drains.

When he comes back into the bedroom she makes that little music sound she makes when it's time. The one they always joke about that sounds like an X-rated movie soundtrack. She stands near the bed and swivels her hips, throwing her long hair back even a little more aggressively than usual so there can be no mistake.

He hovers in the doorway to the bedroom and squints at her.

She makes the sound again, louder, and this time, swivels her rear while looking away.

"Are you crazy?" he asks her, gruffly. "Damn, Susan," he says. He spins on his heel and disappears into the recesses of the house.

And with these five words her sexy mood evaporates like vapor in a desert. Suddenly, her chest throbs. She quickly changes underwear, pulls on sweatpants, and climbs back into bed. *He will never long for me again, I will never be sexy again. He called me crazy. What does that mean? Am I crazy for thinking that all of my sexiness wasn't just in my breasts?* This conviction etches itself into her consciousness and stings.

She forges a brave face for the outside world, but she knows that her sexual side is gone and it haunts her more than fear of recurrence—it is harder than the burn from radiation, and it chips away every time she sees a romantic scene in a movie or watches a couple touching at the real estate office where she works when she feels well enough. She doesn't worry that he'll leave, but she tries to quietly say good-bye to that part of herself.

When I met the couple in my office, the dry had settled around them. It was a few months after treatment had ended. I gently asked each of them to describe their lives since the diagnosis, and on this, they agreed. It had been hell. Neither would talk much, which is uncommon in the beginning of couples therapy. Usually at least one member of a couple has a lot to say. I knew I couldn't barge in with recommendations until we shared a better understanding of their experience, so I went slowly and sent them on date nights to stoke up the romance. I told them that when they were ready, we'd have some honest conversations. Before we could do that, we needed to find a small seed of affection and nurture it awhile.

And then about a month into therapy, while they were both outside raking leaves, he made the sound of that music. It had been more than eight months since they'd been sexual. Eight months of misery. She was angry at first, but then he looked so silly strutting around his rake, his flannel shirt flailing out like a girl's dress. He offered his hand, and, confused, she took it, and then they were back up in the bedroom and it was awkward but OK, even though he didn't seem to know what do with his hands anymore. And after, in the quiet, the anger and hurt lifted like a storm and poured down.

She reminded him of that day when she strutted right there next to the bed, and how horrible she's felt, asexual, and alone. At first she thought he didn't remember—he never remembers the moments that seem so massive to her—but he did, and he listened, to every word, and then, when she was done and it was all out, she half-expected him to bolt from the room and never return.

"Oh no, baby, you got it all wrong," he said finally, taking her hand. "You had those drains and all them stitches. I was scared we'd rip something open. I'd hurt you. And besides, I knew . . . I mean, I was convinced in my heart that you was just doing it for me. . . ." And then he added, "This whole time I thought you hated me, I had no idea why." Looking at this relationship from the outside, their anguish was preventable. These lovers both already had a heaping plate of cancer, they didn't need an additional serving of loneliness, isolation, and self-deprecation. Ultimately, they were fortunate—fortunate they had the courage to ask for help. Fortunate that they'd weathered those eight months without even more serious relationship problems.

In this particular case, I taught them about the benefits and problems with *protection*, a concept we'll cover later in this book. But this is just one of the many predictable challenges cancer whisks into couples' lives.

As I've struggled to understand my own relationships, and those of my patients, I've come to understand how easy it is to lose our mooring in the face of cancer's visit. And how ironic it is that so many of us spin away from the people we love and need most as we venture into the foreign and hostile cancer world.

The stakes are high. The quality of our marriages and relationships appears to impact not only how we feel psychologically but physically, too. Researchers who have followed couples for up to five years—starting with the initial diagnosis—have found that individuals in distressed marriages recover more slowly from cancer treatment and have worse outcomes.[1]

If we scratch, like miners, beneath the surface, we find that we want the same things: To feel that in the abyss, there will be someone there with us. To make us laugh, to hold our hands, and to face the unknown, bravely together.

I wrote this book to help you stand together, shoulder to shoulder, wing to wing, in the doorway of the hostile unknown and emerge at the other end, still deeply in love, intimate, and even . . . when possible . . . frisky.

## Your Tour Guide

I am not happy to have this expertise.

I would trade all the opportunity that has come packaged with my experience for a chemotherapy-free lifetime, but I did not have a choice. I'll bring a few perspectives to this writing. First, and most important, I've played both roles. I've been the supportive spouse and the cancer patient.

For five long years during my early twenties, I battled a resistant, life-threatening lymphatic cancer. In the middle of that struggle I met, dated, and ultimately married my wife, Terry. Against the odds and after a significant amount of treatment, including a failed bone marrow transplant, I was cured, though I wouldn't know it for years. And then, about twelve years later, Terry developed a serious breast cancer that also required significant treatment.

In addition to qualifications as a patient and lover, I'm a Harvard and University of Florida–trained clinical and health psychologist who has researched and worked with couples facing cancer. I also interviewed forty couples for this book—in every couple at least one person had cancer (a few had both had cancer, and one couple had chemotherapy at the same time!). Finally, I teach medical students and residents at a medical school, so I'll bring a few observations about modern medical care, too—in particular, how the care we receive can cause friction between us.

I'm going to try to make this easy and fun to read with plenty of true stories and observations about real people. Along the way, I hope you'll laugh with me a few times, and do some thinking, and in the end, have a thriving relationship.

A few words about organization. This book is written in short, digestible sections that are meant to be mosaic chips that stand on their own, so you can copy just one and share it. Whenever possible I'll ground our discussion in real people's experiences, provide quotes from other couples, and tell stories from our life. Taken together, the mosaic chips will fit together and tell our entire story, as well as provide a guide to most of the issues facing couples when cancer visits.

The first chapter focuses on things to know immediately, just after being diagnosed. Chapter 2 addresses early challenges as we adjust, as a couple, to treatment. The third chapter is designed to help you in interactions with medicine and medical teams. The fourth chapter, and one of the most important, will help you think about your emotional life as a couple during the cancer experience. If you read no other chapter, dig into this one. The fifth chapter focuses on life as we settle into new routines and offers specific advice centered on issues that frequently combust in couples facing cancer. Chapter 6 is about outside relationships and how they can help and harm us. The seventh chapter focuses on sexuality, a key issue for many couples going through cancer. The eighth chapter should help you think about two key issues in relationships during cancer: closeness and dependence. I've also included the ninth chapter, which looks at navigating our relationships at the end of life. Finally, there are a few words about generosity. We'll commence with the key lessons you need at the very beginning, just after being diagnosed. Let's get started.

# 1

# Things to Know Immediately

If you've just been diagnosed, or your spouse has just been diagnosed, I'm sure your head is swimming. For many years I met with newly diagnosed patients, and over time, I developed a "Cancer 101" for couples that consists of three basic parts; all three are in this first chapter. First, I want you to know that even if your relationship isn't perfect, you can still be effective. Second, I'm going to orient you to key relationships in your life now, namely your relationship with your physicians. I'll especially explore how physicians are trained and how this impacts how they communicate. Last, I'll provide some guidelines to help you avoid common conflicts during this period. The chapter has two additional issues that are both important: I'll share some information about the challenges and benefits of doing research on your own; and for those of you of reproductive age, I'll give you some guidance about preserving fertility.

I've got one additional note for you. As you read through this chapter it may feel that I'm making all sorts of recommendations about things you should do early on in your experience when you are both already feeling overwhelmed, afraid, and exhausted. It may be taking enormous effort just to get out of bed, and all of a sudden, you have a new full-time job in addition to all of your old ones. Remember, you only have to do what you have to do today—and if that's too much to think about, just do what you have to do right now. You don't have to cope with the entire cancer experience right now.

## 1-1. Even though our relationships are not perfect, we can forge ourselves into a powerful team.

How do you ever know you are inseparable? We all think we know. We thought we knew before the bug. But we do know now.

—MIKE PROCTOR

When we beat this we're going to be a better married couple.

—TOBIN HODGES

Violins do not start playing when I enter a room, and my hair only rarely flows behind me when I ride bareback through a forest to save my wife from a dragon. Our relationship is not Hollywood perfect. Yours probably isn't either. The good news is that they don't need to be for us to be effective partners.

That said, it will be helpful for us to take a quick peek at our relationships and preferences to help us stave off predictable conflicts that sometimes arise early on in the cancer experience. There are two issues I want you think about now, and both concern how you interact with physicians.

1. You may approach authority differently.
2. Technical expertise and bedside manner may have different levels of importance to the two of you.

Let's start by talking about physicians and their authority. I'm going to share some quick history about physicians and communication with patients to illuminate why some of these discussions aren't optimal.

Cancer surgeries were first described around 1600 B.C.E., or even earlier, on papyri scrolls discovered in the late 1860s in Egypt.[1] We of course don't know if the Egyptian surgeons told their patients the truth about their diagnosis. But at least for the more recent two hundred or so years that physicians have known about cancer, they said little.

In the 1950s, and then again in the 1960s, researchers asked doctors if they told patients when they knew the patient had cancer. The vast majority, over 90 percent, said no. "It would be like putting a person in a concentration camp," one of them wrote.[2]

By the late 1970s, the trend had reversed.[3] By then, there'd been limited success with cancer treatments, the culture around authority had shifted, and physicians started telling patients the truth. Then we moved into an era of legalistic medicine— when physicians were occasionally sued for hiding patients' problems from them—and the pendulum swung dramatically in the other direction. Now physicians often feel obligated to share any potential bad outcome—including obscure side effects of necessary medications.

So if you think about it, modern physicians have only thirty or so years of experience sharing the truth with patients. And there is no gold standard for how physicians should tell patients that they have cancer.

I received "big" bad news three times, and along the way there were many more smaller bits of bad news. And each time, the physicians did the task differently. Most physicians muddle through, sharing statistics and treatment options and explaining in great detail why they know it's cancer and not something else.

Personally, I like the simple approach where they say what's wrong and discuss a potential plan. But most of them talk quite a bit. I suspect they muddle through partially because we teachers in medical schools have only been asking young physicians to practice this art for a short time.

Here's an example of muddling: Some of them try to tell us there's good news and bad news. For example, the good news is that we have terrific parking near the chemotherapy suites. The bad news is that you're going to need it! Others play professor, drawing cells on the crinkly white paper while gesturing and using words like multiplication rates, as if we are all fascinated in the same way they are by the science of it all. Finally, many physicians are still learning how to balance attention to the electronics that have invaded clinic rooms with attention to the patient. Some of them spend too much time looking at their computers, focused only on entering our information so that the electronic record will be complete.

Of course, what we want in these situations is for the physician to say that he or she has a great plan of attack and it will include X, Y, and Z. And then we want them to look at us squarely in our faces and say, "I'm so sorry the news is bad, but I will not rest until I've done everything in my power to ensure your survival. I'll be here with you every step of the way."

And we want them to say these things while sitting down and looking at us. Then we want them to ask us if we have questions. And then to patiently and thoughtfully answer those questions.

## The Physician Side of the Equation

> Some people put their doctors up on some sort of pedestal, sort of like some people do their ministers. They are people just like we are, and they just happen to be doctors. I kept pushing and pushing and pushing. If I would not have I don't believe my husband would be alive today.
>
> —LINDA SPENCE

Often physicians schedule their returning patients every fifteen minutes, with new patients getting a half hour or a little longer. If a patient visit scheduled early in the day stretches to be longer than its allotted fifteen minutes—say because of a series of complex problems or because an unscheduled patient has a crisis and needs to be seen—the rest of the day's schedule can be thrown off entirely. And two early complex patients? Well, forget it. Everyone will be waiting. This is the most common complaint about physicians, but it is not the only one.

Recent surveys produced by the Arnold P. Gold Foundation (who queried six hundred patients across the country, including a number who were themselves medical professionals) revealed that 70 percent of patients feel they regularly wait too long to see their physician, 43 percent felt they had too little opportunity to discuss serious concerns, and 47 percent felt that their physicians often seemed rushed. Smaller percentages had dealt with more severe problems, including physicians who were distracted by simultaneously entering notes while tending to the patient (18 percent), physicians being rude or condescending (20 percent), and those who used confusing medical terms (7 percent).[4]

Studies that have tape-recorded conversations between oncologists and patients and then carefully examined them for the presence of patient emotion and oncologist empathy have found that oncologists only respond to patients' emotional expressions with empathy about one-fifth of the time.[5]

We can see, then, that there is a very high likelihood that we will spend significant time waiting. And there is the possibility that we will run into a condescending physician. And it's likely that if we express our sadness or fears, the doctor will, well, just sit or stand there.

Unfortunately many of us approach meetings with physicians in the same way we approach bringing a broken appliance to a repairman. When I was a child, my family lived across the street from Victor Spachek, a Czechoslovakian immigrant who fixed televisions out of his garage. My father occasionally carried our wounded Zenith across the street and would say, "Vic, I dunno. It's broken." And Vic would nod soberly and take the patient from my father. A few days later the television would be back. Just like that.

But physicians are not television repairmen. Even if we are passive people, cancer often requires us to be active participants in our own care. We may have to manage complex medication regimens, distinguish common treatment side effects from those that are dangerous, and communicate clearly to improve our comfort during treatments.

We may also need to speak up if we have been kept waiting for a long time and assertively address those less common physicians who are condescending. This requires that we have some skills at a time when we often feel vulnerable and depleted.

You will do better as a couple if you become a team. That is, whenever you meet with the physician, you will each have a job. Perhaps one of you will ask the questions first, while the other writes down the answers. And then switch. Both of you may have legitimate questions to ask.

Important information is shared at early visits, such as whom the physician wants us to consult next, what kind of information is still needed to decide the staging of the illness (how far it's progressed)—which will influence treatment options—or what the treatment options might be. And we're being asked to remember that information when it feels like the roof has blown away, leaving behind cracked timber and howling wind. It can be enormously difficult to concentrate.

## The Patient Side of the Equation

First of all we're not medical people. You hear all these big terms, you hear all this medical language, you're overwhelmed.

—DAVID MILSON

Some couples have conflicts early when they disagree about how to respond to a physician, nurse, or other key health professional. Consider Gerry. He noted that when he was with his wife's radiation oncologist, the man was always late and seemed rushed—so Gerry asked him why. "Doc, gotta ask, we come in here, and every time Alice sees you there's no time to ask even a single question. What's the story?"

He told me, "Here's the difference between me and my wife. If she goes to a restaurant and the waiter brings the wrong meal, she'll eat it. I won't." But from Alice's perspective, her husband was unnecessarily antagonizing the very people on whom her life depended. And she wanted them to like her. She felt like she was in the ocean and that her husband was angering the only people who had a life raft. "So what if they're late or don't talk much?" she said.

I understand both perspectives. Early on in my cancer experience I remember trying to engage my physician. There was a part of me that believed that if my doctors cared about me more than the other patients, they would go the extra mile to make sure I survived. Perhaps they'd call the international experts to consult, mull over my laboratory reports late at night and on weekends, and call me a few times an hour to see how I was doing. I couldn't bake, sew, or provide other delectables, so I tried to be funny and upbeat—even entertaining.

And on the other side, when I was a spouse, I wanted Terry to be treated well. And perhaps I couldn't do anything to fight the cancer, but I could make sure that no one treated her badly. On a number of occasions I spoke up. I was direct with physicians when they didn't treat her well and indignant when she was made to wait for what I perceived to be too long.

There's a balance to find here. We don't want to be known in medical environments as entitled brats and, at the same time, we don't want to get run over or suffer from carelessness because we didn't speak up.

I *have* seen patients who were entitled and demanding. Once, during my fellowship in a Boston hospital, an angry oncologist who had received a number of calls about trivial issues asked me to work with a patient and her family. The oncologist said, "These people think our unit is a hotel. Please remind them that it's more like a prison."

The tricky part for couples is when these two perspectives collide: when one member of the couple wants the medical teams to like him or her so much that it feels to them like a high-pressure popularity contest, and the other treats the health professionals like unloved employees.

I want you to have two tools in your couple's toolbox. I want you to treat health professionals like the overworked, well-intentioned, and hard-working people they are most of the time—and speak up when important needs are going unaddressed. We'll address the need for caregivers to advocate for their spouses in more detail later, but for now, I want you to decide: Who will speak up if you are left in the waiting room for an hour? Which one of you will ask for more time with the physician or nurse if you have unanswered questions? Who will write things down or record them? I also want you to ask: Under what circumstances should we contact the medical team between visits?

I also want you to decide which of you will speak up if you happen to run into one of those condescending physicians. And less dramatically, which of you will be assertive if your questions aren't being answered sufficiently, or if the doctor is giving the electronic medical record more attention than you.

I want you to have these conversations not only for now but for the long-term, because it sets you up as a functional team.

Also: Recognize that both of these approaches are valid. It's reasonable to want to be liked when your life depends on these professionals, and reasonable to want to protect and stand up for yourselves. Let's turn now to a common tension among couples: navigating decisions about whom we put our trust in.

## 1-2. The person with the body gets to decide if the doc is a "match."

If you are not comfortable asking the people in the room anything, then they are not the right people even if they may be the best at what they do.

—ROSS KING

Sometimes I'll ask David to come in with me and he'll come in and he'll sit very quietly. He'll have that pleasant, assuring look on his face. There are other times when I won't want him [in there with the doctors] and he never questions that. He'll never say, Why did you not want me to go in this time, why did you want to go in this alone and not have me come in? He doesn't do it.

—SANDRA WILKERSON

In the 1800s the busiest physicians typically saw only eight patients per day, making house calls. In the 1930s, four out of ten patient-physician contacts were still house calls,[6] and even in 1950, the average length of stay in some hospitals was well more than twenty days.[7] You can see that physicians used to spend considerable time with patients.

Now the average length of stay in a hospital is less than five days,[8] and it's only that long because some people stay in hospital intensive care units for months, pulling up the average. In addition, our outpatient visits are shorter than they were for the generations that came before us, with the average face-to-face time with a physician being well less than ten minutes (though oncologists spend considerably more than this—about nineteen minutes, on average).[9]

Put simply, we don't get much time with physicians. And when we do, it can feel pressured. (It's also true that in at least a third of physician visits, physicians interrupt patients early in the conversation—but while this has been widely quoted, the data actually reveal that when physicians interrupt, they tend to get it right. It's when they seem withdrawn that we tend to disagree with them about the usefulness of the meeting.)

One of the frustrating truths about being a patient is that it's incredibly difficult to tell how technically competent a physician is from watching and listening. It was difficult for us, and my wife is an oncology nurse practitioner!

We need physicians who have great bedside manner and great technical competence when we face cancer. I have colleagues in integrative medicine who believe that technical competence cannot be divorced from bedside manner, because a physician with good bedside manner can elicit more information from a patient—but in cancer, it is most important to have docs who are up-to-date on the latest data, carefully study a patient's response to treatments like chemotherapy, and who think carefully through treatment options.

Here's the problem: It's easy to mistake great bedside manner for great technical competence. We can almost always tell how good their bedside manner is, because we feel it in our guts. But for technical competence, we tend to rely on indicators of competence that may or may not be reliable. These indicators include things such as where they practice, what we've heard about them, and even how fancy the waiting room appears. But none of these is necessarily predictive of how hard they will work if our situation is complex, or how creative or dedicated they are.

In many ways, choosing a physician or practice is an educated act of faith. As such, it's common for couples to disagree about the quality of a given physician—because to an extent, we're both guessing.

Our physicians should be able to tell us how many other patients with similar circumstances they've treated, the data they are relying on to make their decisions, and whether they are willing to consult with other physicians to assist us. These are key indicators of quality.

It's essential that the patient feel confident in his or her physician, and this is a decision that is deeply personal and may require that the spouse be supportive even when they disagree. Ultimately, the person with the body gets to choose the physician.

## 1-3. The person with the body gets to make the major decisions about his or her body.

From the very beginning, my husband supported the idea of mastectomy. I was not able to have immediate reconstruction due to the pregnancy, so basically I was left with a growing lactating breast that we fondly referred to as "Wanda the Wonder Tit" and a severely deformed, almost concave, side, and a growing belly. I had to wear a whole series of prostheses in order to match Wanda, who seemed to be growing at a record rate. My husband always told me how beautiful he thought I was. I gave birth to my son via C-section (yet another scar to add to my collection) and three weeks later started the first of four rounds of Adriamyacin/Cytoxan chemo. After the first round, he shaved my head, first into a Mohawk and then clean off. I was sad and worried, but he never skipped a beat both emotionally and physically. He never shied away from touching my deformed side during lovemaking.

—LAUREN STONE

So then the results come in, and often there are some decisions to make. Some couples do this quite well. They systematically look over the options, talk about them, and come to an agreement relatively quickly. In many situations, the options are also not equal, and the vast majority of us would make the same decision. But in some illnesses—particularly breast and prostate cancer—there are some choices with different consequences.

And here's the reality. One of you may be making decisions that will impact both of you. In prostate cancer, for example, there are a variety of decisions to make about the type of surgery to have (if any), and they have different side-effect profiles—with one common option being more likely to render a patient impotent, and the other option more likely to result in leaking urine. Or there may be questions about how aggressive to be. In breast cancer, for example, many patients now get double mastectomies even when only one breast is involved, while other patients prefer to have the most minimal surgery, understanding that the risk of recurrence is greater.

Consider one of our interactions. In Terry's case, the tumor was finger-thin and at least four centimeters long. And the cells had crawled out of the breast and into the lymph nodes beneath her arm. She wanted both of her breasts off. Now.

"Why both?" I asked.

"Why not?" she said.

"But that one hasn't done anything wrong," I said, pointing vaguely at her left side.

She glowered. "And I'm having the ovaries out; my cancer is fed by estrogen, so out they go."

Terry's breasts had surprised me during our time together. They started out modest, and in my naiveté, I didn't realize that over a lifetime breasts change size. During the high doses of estrogen she imbibed during our infertility adventures they grew denser and larger. Pert, even. She could fill a large bathing suit top with some to spare. And then when she got pregnant they grew again, rounder and even larger. Suddenly she had cleavage, which entertained her, and needed new bras and a host of other lotions, potions, tinctures, and creams to cope with challenges of breast-feeding.

On more than one occasion I enjoyed looking down her shirt when she leaned over to pick up Alexandra, and I admit to coming up behind her and cupping her in my hands before getting smacked.

So when she was diagnosed, I had opinions. I liked her breasts. And having one's ovaries out seemed severe, too. She was going to leap into menopause. But for once, I muzzled my opinions. It was, after all, her body. Her survival. And just like I had once decided that I wanted more treatment even when things looked bleak, it was her call to make.

So if you're the partner, your job is to help the patient get the best information available, and then chime in if asked. But most of all, be supportive. *This is true even though partners will have to live with these decisions, too.* I suggest you say, "I'll support and love you no matter which decision you make." For patients: make the decision that you feel most comfortable with—not the one that will be most pleasing to your partner. Not making the best decision for you can lead to resentment later, and this can be lethal for the relationship.

## 1-4. Do responsible research early.

When I relapsed after a bone marrow transplant, my situation looked grim. Unlike four years before, when physicians shared that my probability of five-year survival was at least 70 percent, now my doctor cast about for words, avoiding my eyes. This was, in fact, my second relapse, and I knew my body was tired from all of the heavy treatment.

Right between my collarbones, an inch beneath my Adam's apple, I could feel the new tumor. It was fixed and dense, like tire rubber. My oncologist felt it, and one of his eyelids blinked repeatedly. He rubbed the bridge of his nose, bowed his head, and washed his hands, and then sat on the stool next to us. He looked down and said that perhaps we should consider the difficult question of whether we wanted to continue treatments given the situation.

We left his office devastated.

But the next day Terry called a friend, an oncologist at the hospital, and asked what he knew about Hodgkin's disease. Who are the best physicians in the world? We didn't have the Internet—it was 1990—but we did have computer-based science search engines. While my fiancée called every person she could think of to ask, I went to the library and looked up original articles on Hodgkin's lymphoma and began assembling a list of the physician-authors who were writing scientific articles about my disease.

Together, we generated the names of three people whom we felt were the national experts. They were in Chicago, Nebraska, and Palo Alto, California. I decided to call them. I felt a little like a telemarketer, cold-calling physicians, but my fear of dying was energizing—and what did I have to lose? In the worst case, they wouldn't talk with me. But with some persistence over a week, I managed to get all three of them on the phone.

The first two concurred with my local physician and gently suggested that more treatment was futile. The third, only slightly irritated that I'd called him during his quiet lab time before work (I'd forgotten that little detail about time zones), said, "Yes. Well. Sorry about your circumstance. So. Call our clinic. My clinic days for new patients are Wednesdays. Make an appointment. Bring every record you have. Oh, and wait to call for a few hours, they aren't open until eight our time, understand?"

As it turned out, that persistence would be rewarded a thousandfold.

In most cases, you will not need to do this kind of aggressive research. Most of our cases are common and physicians have well-researched protocols for applying them. But in some cases, when our circumstance is rare or dire, it makes sense to go to the best.

I want you to find the best physicians in your area if your disease is common, and consult the best physicians in the nation if your illness is uncommon or your situation seems dire. You have resources you may not have considered, including the Internet and other patients. PUBMED is a search engine at the Institute of Medicine that you can find using any computer connected to the Internet. It is a central clearinghouse for scientific articles. You don't need to understand the science to study the names of the individuals doing research. You can then search the institutions where they are to learn if they see patients. Don't be afraid to make phone calls. A little additional research can save our lives.

## 1-5. There may be five ways to kill a man, but there are a thousand ways to freak yourselves out on the Internet. Understand which information to get on the Internet.

Try NOT to get super-consumed with the diagnosis; don't try to research on the Internet everything that it took many, many years for oncologists to learn.

—Deborah Kennedy

He didn't want to hear some of the bad news. But he did want to know what was going on. So I could do the research. I filtered through and told him what he needed to know but not all of the different statistics.

—Helen Kelley

I've just suggested that doing research can be helpful. In my opinion, doing research is good for finding the right people; it's much harder to find the right procedures or weigh one treatment against another.

Let's talk about how to use, and not use, the Internet. Roughly 85 percent of people are "information seeking," and in a given year, roughly 50 percent of American adults seek information about personal health concerns with most using the Internet.[10] That is, when faced with a novel threatening situation, like cancer, they want information. During my travels as a psychologist, I've met some of the people in the other 15 percent. They tended to be more religious and, specifically, trust that a higher power was looking out for them and would make information available when it was necessary. Frankly, I envied them, but my mind doesn't operate like this (and if you're reading this, it's likely your mind doesn't work that way either).

After meeting with Terry's surgeon we drove home. I raced to the computer and looked up breast cancer. In the case of my cancer, Hodgkin's disease, the data had been relatively straightforward. There are four subtypes, and then the question of how advanced it had gotten. I'd had the most popular form (woo hoo!). Once I knew that, I could look up my prognosis.

With Terry's breast cancer, the situation was more complex. First, there's the question of how large the tumor was and how far it had crawled. We knew the sample the surgeon had taken had been cancerous, but not its size. We didn't yet know if the tumor had managed to get out of the breast and into the lymph nodes. Nor did we know what fueled the tumors. Sometimes hormones fuel breast cancer, but there are other factors too. And then there's the multiplication rate, or how many of the cells are aggressive, and margins and protein expression and then even these new experimental factors. It was dizzying.

And then one of the articles I found referred to cancer as the second leading cause of death in women. (Heart disease is "number one.")

My head nearly exploded.

I am a well-educated person. I know how to use major medical search engines, I regularly read *Sciencedaily* online, which summarizes major scientific articles and sometimes even interviews the researchers. Not to mention a few newspapers and Internet mailing lists. And then there are the various sites that summarize diseases for laypeople.

It is tempting to want to know everything there is to know about the new invader in our lives, particularly when there are decisions to make, but trying to simulate an education in oncology is futile, because the Internet is a three-car garage stuffed by hoarders. There's valuable stuff in there, but if you don't know where to look you can spend all your time clearing off rodent droppings and chewed Beanie Babies.

And then, what are you going to do with prognostic information once you have it? Does it really make anything more predictable? Or will the numbers just rattle around in your head at three A.M.? The reality is, either our lives are 100 percent going to be shortened by the disease, or 100 percent not. And given that I had survived a disease after having a poor chance of survival, I should have known better. In my case, when I did finally see the international expert on Hodgkin's disease, he looked at all of my scans. He pulled a chair up to mine, put a hand on my shoulder, and looked me right in the eyes. He said, "I don't think I can cure you, but I'll try."

Yet, with Terry's disease, I immediately pored over data from Web sites like "cancerwillkillyou.com." I was immediately overwhelmed by it all. When I should have been focusing on Terry and making her waiting time better, instead I pressed my face against glass of the worst possible outcomes. The reality is, it's impossible to quickly digest all of the information that would make you an oncologist fast enough to be helpful to yourself, and the emotional consequences of having just enough information to be dangerous to yourself and others can be profound.

I want you to use the Internet and other information resources to find good doctors or learn about side effects of treatments. The Internet will be useful for many things, but it is not the place to go looking for the ultimate truth about our future. Once you have your plan and understand the treatment, stay away from searches with words like "survival," "prognosis," and "death rate." Remember: survival percentages apply to large groups of people (usually even data being published now are already old) and there is no way to tell which of those numbers applies to you.

Studies have shown that we also often go to the Internet when we are dissatisfied with the communication we've had with health professionals.[11] Sometimes this is because we were unable to concentrate when we had the focused attention of health professionals; sometimes this occurs when we feel our health professionals are not communicating well. We also go when we've had a disagreement with our spouse over something a health professional said. In general, the Internet is a great place to connect with other survivors and to learn skills and technical information. It's a lousy place to find an oracle.

There are also Internet mailing lists. Anyone with an e-mail address can subscribe to a mailing list focused on a specific type of cancer or problem. These are also sometimes called listserves. The Association of Cancer Online Resources (ACOR) sponsors a number of moderated listserves where survivors offer information and emotional support to other survivors. Studies of these listserves show that survivors do find what they are seeking on these lists.[12] The advantage of listserves is that subscribers have access to the wisdom of many patients, and because the messages are filtered by a moderator, they tend to stay on-topic, so the drivel-to-substance ratio is favorable.

Frequently, it is logistics that prevents us from doing research or traveling to consult other physicians. It can feel terribly overwhelming to do additional research when you already feel depleted. And yet, this is the time when the extra effort is rewarded.

Work as a team to address these logistical challenges. Logistics tend to fall into a few categories: calling people you don't know to get information or set up appointments; making travel plans including flights, coverage for children, parents, pets, plants, and other household needs; financial decisions; and interacting with coworkers to get coverage at work.

Start with a list and work your way down, assigning jobs to the person most capable of getting any given task done efficiently. If possible, enlist your closest friends or family to help with tasks they can accomplish. Often people in your network may want to assist you but have little idea how—this is a time to assign specific tasks to people to help you get to the best medical people available.

Here's an additional piece of information. There is a national trend developing now in academic cancer centers where physicians from different specialties who work on the same illnesses are starting to share clinic space in order to learn from one another's experiences and better address patient needs. This has long been true of breast cancer, but now it is also developing in prostate, skin, lung, and a variety of other cancers. If possible, try to be seen in these centers, as I suspect the treatment is better because those doctors communicate more regularly. It is also usually far more convenient. These clinics are often called "specialty clinics" or "medical homes."

While making numerous logistical decisions and simultaneously feeling occasionally as if one's head is going to explode from the stress, it is natural to make some mistakes. You may need to check things twice and be extra careful with phone numbers, dates, locations, and details.

## 1-6. If you are a couple of reproductive age, advances in fertility preservation may surprise you. Preserve fertility options.

We don't know if I'm human because I was made in a test tube in a laboratory.

—ALEXANDRA SHAPIRO (announced to her first-grade class)

Of the 1.5 million of us diagnosed with cancer every year, about 10 percent are in our reproductive years.[13] It is very difficult to simultaneously face a cancer diagnosis and consider all of the long-term consequences of treatment, but for a moment, let's focus on fertility options.

I was diagnosed with cancer when I was twenty years old and started chemotherapy, which rendered me sterile, only a few weeks after the diagnosis. But I have two biological children—girls—because my mother happened to speak to another patient's mother and learned about sperm banking, which I did prior to starting treatment. For men, I strongly recommend banking sperm.

Women also have a number of options. The most common is delaying treatment to have one cycle of hormone stimulation followed by the harvesting of eggs, fertilization of eggs, and preservation of the oocyte or embryos. In addition, a small number of women have now also successfully had ovarian tissue removed, had chemotherapy, then had the tissue reimplanted, generated eggs, become pregnant, and successfully given birth.[14] Young girls are also having eggs removed and stored now.

In some situations, treatment can also be tailored to preserve fertility for patients with lower-risk disease. For example, reducing radiation dosage for patients with low-risk Hodgkin's disease and forgoing alkylating chemotherapy drugs for patients with breast cancer can also be negotiated.

Here's the take-home message. Speaking with our oncologists and other health professionals about the preservation of fertility is important, because many health professionals are so distracted by treating the disease that they forget to address this critical issue with us. Data suggest that many oncologists are still not referring patients to reproductive specialists, even though most want to follow the guidelines established in 2007 by the American Society of Clinical Oncology. These guidelines dictate that all patients of reproductive age should be told about the risks of infertility following cancer treatments. In fact, most physicians do not discuss fertility preservation with newly diagnosed cancer patients, and when they don't, it's often because of their own personal discomfort.[15] And when they do speak to patients, they often don't know the latest information. This is somewhat understandable—the field is moving quickly—but it's probably also true that oncologists think of fertility as belonging to gynecologists and reproductive endocrinologists.

I advise you to check the Web site "Fertile Hope" (www.fertile hope.org). Fertile Hope is a nonprofit recently acquired by the Lance Armstrong Foundation, and it supports and studies the newest fertility options for cancer patients. There is also a fairly new consortium of fertility specialists around the country who are working together to study new methods to preserve fertility. Called the Oncofertility Consortium, they have a Web site based at Northwestern University in Chicago (http://oncofertility .northwestern.edu).

Now let's turn to a complex fertility issue. Sometimes a cancer diagnosis stimulates complex conversations about the future. This is especially common in couples who are very close but not quite ready to think about having children. I saw one young unmarried couple who had not yet talked about having children but suddenly had to face complex decisions: Should she freeze only her eggs? Should they freeze embryos? They were deeply in love but had not talked about marriage yet; they'd only been together for eighteen months.

She was intensely anxious because she wanted to preserve her fertility, but the implications of any action she took frightened her. If she elected to freeze only her eggs, she might communicate to her boyfriend that she was planning for the deterioration of their relationship. If she elected to freeze embryos, she'd feel she was rushing the relationship, and if they didn't stay together, she'd be left having to discard the embryos, a stressful experience regardless of one's position on the abortion debate.

I urged her, and urge you, to preserve as many of your options as is possible. In her case, that meant postponing treatment long enough so that she could freeze some embryos fertilized by her boyfriend and some of her eggs.

It is absolutely true that this "rushed" her relationship in that she and her boyfriend had to discuss their situation and the possibility of their wanting to have children together someday. They also discussed the possibility of the relationship not working out. It was, to say the least, an awkward and somewhat painful discussion, but she did both and was happy to discover that he was enthusiastic about freezing embryos.

Clearly, there are some deeply personal decisions to make here. Patients who feel that a fertilized embryo is a human life may not be able to make peace with the decision if they do not ultimately use the embryos. For those patients, the risk of infertility is likely more palatable than ultimately discarding frozen embryos.

The challenge here is that many of these discussions are made while the shock of the diagnosis still hangs in the air. Because advances happen quickly, consult a reproductive endocrinologist to learn more. It is likely that your oncologist will not be completely up-to-date. If you have access to many reproductive endocrinologists, such as in major metropolitan areas, you can also learn about success rates of various clinics by consulting the Web site of the Society for Assisted Reproductive Endocrinology (SART). The Web site allows searchers to find a clinic based on geographical location, and it offers success rates from each clinic, listed as ART data reports. These publicly accessible reports provide each center's success rates using various technologies and techniques. For example, you can find data such as the percentage of cycles resulting in live births and how many embryos they tend to transfer. Ideally, you will talk to these centers about your options for preserving reproduction before you start treatment.

## 1-7. Chances are, you can withstand more than you expect. So can your spouse.

I am very squeamish. He always cleaned up when the kids threw up. I can't stand anything like that. I can't stand blood, I can't stand anything gross. My taking care of the many things that I've taken care of, I do not understand to this day how I did it. I just did it. I am so shocked that I didn't pass out and fall on the floor.

—LINDA SPENCE

I'm a lot stronger than a lot of people thought I was. Or even me, I guess.

—RHONDA T.

I am not normally this strong person. I've had to turn into this person. People keep saying, "Are you OK?" I really am. I'm OK because I know it's going to be OK. I can't sit and be down about it. It's not going to do any good. What good is it going to do him if he sees me all down about it?

—Valree Milson

Before concluding the very first chapter, I wanted to share something I've seen again and again, that I hope you find comforting. One of the impressive things we often learn about ourselves during the cancer experience is that we are more resilient than we expect. Psychological study of people under enormous stress reveals that most of us have reserves and capabilities we don't fully understand until we are forced to draw on them. This has been found of concentration camp inmates, victims of war, and survivors of tragedies such as car accidents or the sudden loss of family members.

My clinical work and interviews with numerous couples echoed these findings. Many patients and spouses told me, "Well, I love her, so I did it." A few spouses also told me, "I've always wondered how I'd be in this situation. I wanted to know that I was the type of person who could handle it, so I did." Not that many of these experiences aren't still unpleasant—they are—it's just that our affection for one another can fuel us far more than we expect.

Patients and their lovers shared with me that they've discovered that they have the capability to deal with a plethora of unexpected challenges. They changed colostomy bags, helped one another with toileting, changed crusty bandages, and dealt with the full spectrum of gross things that can emerge from a human body. Not that you're definitely going to have do those things—but if you do, you may be pleased to discover that you are capable of adjusting to these unpleasantries.

Psychologically, my patients and the people I interviewed coped with fierce disappointments and discovered greater patience and—for many—greater assertiveness. A number of spouses told me that they generally approach authority with deference, but when it came to their lover being ill, they learned that they could be a "yappy junkyard dog" as one spouse put it. They learned to set limits with unhelpful family members, nurture even when they felt depleted, and find some comfort for themselves. These are just a few of the themes we'll turn to in the next chapter, which focuses on navigating our relationships successfully through the early phases of the experience.

# 2

# Navigating Your Relationship through Early Challenges

Cancer is complex psychologically because it's like a tremor that rattles our walls and finds the fault lines that already existed. If we're not careful, it reaches into our relationships and drags out these subtle differences and magnifies them.

Remember the first couple at the beginning of this book? Susan and her husband were both deeply hurt when Susan tried to initiate sex soon after her surgery. You'll recall that he found her back in the bedroom and rejected her swiveling hips. As I learned more, I discovered that well before cancer there was a common tension in their relationship: she resented how often he wanted to have sex, and sometimes after they had sex, she'd make comments revealing that she disliked feeling pressured. While this was an aspect of their marriage they were normally able to manage, the presence of cancer elevated their emotions beyond what was healthy.

In this chapter, I'll be asking you to think about the fault lines in your relationship—the subtle and maybe not so subtle tensions that exist between the two of you—so that we can help you evade common conflicts and form a powerful partnership. Let's turn to some of the common fault lines that get rattled in those early moments, when the sirens of diagnosis are still wailing in our minds. I'm going to share a number of common issues I've seen that lead to conflicts or other relationship problems.

## 2-1. Cancer is a new experience. Tolerate not being great at it right away. Tolerate your spouse not being great at it either.

I get really mad and yell or turn around and won't talk. My husband is a much nicer arguer.

—HELEN KELLEY

I am passive-aggressive.

—RICHARD KELLEY

I saw one couple who had a vicious fight because while she was getting chemotherapy for the first time at a large teaching hospital, her husband parked the car in the wrong place. He parked much farther away, in the usual patient parking lot, instead of in the special cancer parking lot that was closer and easier to navigate.

He had failed to pay attention when the receptionist told him on the phone that he should park in the special lot. As a result, his wife had to wait an extra twenty minutes after chemotherapy while he fetched the vehicle, waited in line to pay to leave, and then circled the hospital to get back to the cancer center exit.

There is no doubt that waiting to get home after chemotherapy is hard. After chemo we crave the safety and comfort of our own environment. And there is no doubt that he should have been paying closer attention to the instructions. In her mind, this wasn't just a parking error. He had demonstrated that in the midst of the largest crisis of their lives, he would not be up to the challenge. He was going to be a space cadet, and she was going to have to manage not only the cancer but also his lame ability to be helpful when she needed him most. This was a looming catastrophe.

In his mind, he was doing the best he could—he'd already negotiated with his usually unforgiving boss to get time off regularly during the six months of chemotherapy, he'd serviced the Honda to make sure they wouldn't have car troubles on a treatment day, and he sat quietly with her—like she wanted—during the ninety-minute treatment without once checking his cell phone for work e-mails.

Meanwhile, his head was spinning with all sorts of fears of chemo—would she have one of the many horrible but rare side effects listed in the pamphlet they'd received from the nurses? He was also worried that he might not keep his job if the business continued to deteriorate and he was the employee out all the time. So it was true that he was distracted when they talked about where to park, but this hardly represented a likely failure in his ability to stand with her during the crisis. Instead, it was just a rookie mistake.

Cancer requires a whole new set of skills at a time when most of us are depleted, distracted, and scared. And when we are stressed we do silly things like lose our purses, leave groceries sitting on the trunk of the car, and park in the wrong places.

This doesn't mean that we won't be helpful long-term in the face of a crisis.

Instead of berating our partners, expect a few rookie mistakes from both of you and tolerate them. You will both get better at this. And how we behave at the beginning is not, actually, a good predictor of how we will behave later. So go easy on your spouse. Go easy on yourself. Stay off the generalization train.

## 2-2. For partners: In the beginning, tell him or her that you love them. A lot. And show it.

One very funny breast cancer story was when my best friend got married at the Ocean Club in the Bahamas. My son was almost five months old and we left him with my mother in New Jersey. I had just finished chemo and had a slight film of hair covering my head. I brought my wig and a myriad of prostheses to cover all events—swimming, formal wear, casual wear, and so on. Anyway, my husband and my best friend urged me not to wear my wig. So since it was so hot, I obliged. I was dubbed by all wedding guests "the bald chick," but I found the whole experience very liberating. We went on to have a wonderful six-day vacation but were very excited to get home to our baby.

Due to a very long line at the provincial airport in Nassau, we almost missed the plane. My husband grabbed my carry-on so we could run to the gate. This was post–September 11th, so they were arbitrarily detaining passengers for a more thorough search. I was let on the plane but my husband was detained with my carry-on containing three fake boobs and a wig. By the time he made it to our seats, he told me that I had just witnessed the greatest act of love that he could ever show me. I am sure the people in the Bahamas thought they had a cross-dresser on their hands. We laughed so hard.

—LAUREN STONE

He hugged me a lot.

—PRISCILLA LABONTE

When Terry and I were first dating, and then getting serious, in those early days of early love's ether, Terry wanted to hear me say "I love you." I wanted to hear her say it, too.

*Yes, I love you, let me tell you how many ways and you are the love of my life.* Smooch Smooch SMOOCH. And on and on and on.

Then, as time went on, what she really wanted—and the best way for me to show my love—was to take out the trash and get my dishes into the dishwasher. I could say "I love you" all the time, but if I didn't get the trash down to the street without being reminded, what she heard was, "If I could get away with it I'd sell you for your kidneys."

And I knew she loved me when she put a T-shirt under my pillow. I hate light when I'm sleeping, and I use the T-shirts to cover my face. She makes the beds in the morning, and she slips a T-shirt under the pillow for me. When I find one there at night, I think, "Ah, she loves me."

And usually, when I've done something to tick her off, there's no T-shirt under my pillow. She "forgets." And if I'm being completely honest, I sometimes space on taking the trash out to the street when I'm angry at her and then she has to remind me. So you can see the problem here, coming down the pike. If one of us gets ill and can't do the thing that communicates our love to the other, we could be set up for a problem. Even though we know it's the illness, on a more primitive level, we still often make that mistake of confusing illness-induced inability for a lack of love.

In the face of cancer, Terry needed to hear the words again. A lot. I love you. *And* she wanted me to take the trash down to the street on time and without being reminded and get my dishes into the dishwasher.

When Terry was being diagnosed, she stopped doing certain things around the house. At first, when I didn't find a T-shirt beneath the pillow, it was easy for me to think, *Hey, she's forgotten about me* or *What did I do wrong?* or more dangerous, *She doesn't love me anymore.*

For some couples, this is particularly true of meals. Suddenly, Mom, who has always made dinner, is in bed and tells everyone, "There's food in there, you're on your own." For some of us, the kitchen is a foreign place with secret formulas and unknown elaborate processes for turning raw ingredients into edible sustenance. And if we do the wrong thing there are germs and mold and uncooked food—or worse, fire! *If she loved me, she'd help me in here* is a dangerous place to go.

Touch is also important. Most couples have established a level of nonsexual touch from "we touch one another whenever we're near the other person" to "we never touch." I want you to increase your level of touch by one notch—I'm referring here to those moments when both of you are in the kitchen or bath or pass in the hall—the soft nonsexual touch on the arm or shoulder can be a soothing balm when we feel vulnerable.

Check out these research findings. When teachers touch students, those students are almost twice as likely to volunteer as other students.[1] Patients touched by doctors perceive that their visits lasted twice as long as untouched patients. And when loved ones massage patients, there are improvements in depression and pain perceptions.[2] All from a little touch! There's even evidence that athletes who touch teammates regularly have more success. When we feel vulnerable, touch can be a magic soothing balm.[3]

Now, when the winds of illness are blowing through our homes, it's essential that we express our love out loud and not allow our changed roles to speak for us. Even those of us who aren't so great at expressing ourselves need to step up and speak up. Tell the other that you love them. Whenever we can, we also show them.

## 2-3. Don't talk about your relationships, buy a house, or adopt a new child (or a ferret) while waiting for the results of scans, biopsies, or other tests.

I decided that I was finally going to confront my boss about how badly I'd been treated. I mean, this had been building for a while, but I'd never seen it quite this way before. I almost marched into his office and really let him have it, but my wife said I should calm down, and I yelled at her, too. Funny, after we got the results from my biopsy I was devastated but wasn't angry at my boss anymore. Well, I was still a little angry, but nothing like that, you know?

—ANONYMOUS MAN

Waiting for results of biopsies, scans, and bloodwork can drag us into a time warp where everything slows. Ten minutes can feel like ten hours.

Unfortunately, most diagnoses are a process. First, we discover that something is there that shouldn't be. After the shock of bad news, we often face a trickle of more bloodwork, biopsies, or scans. Each of these can paint a new corner of the diagnostic picture. And usually, those results don't come back nearly as quickly as we would like.

Consider the average X-ray. In most radiology departments, radiologists try to "turn around" every X-ray within forty-eight hours. But some take longer. And when I say "turn around," I mean that it takes that long for the radiologist to read and dictate a paragraph about the scan. Then the report needs to be read by the nurse or physician in the office where you were seen, and then you need to be notified. For bloodwork, the range is vast— from an hour if the work is ordered emergently in some places, to over five days if it lands behind a bunch of other urgent work, say from the emergency room.

While the diagnosis is urgent to us, the reality is that for most cancers it's not considered as medically urgent as, say, a suicide attempt in which someone has swallowed a huge number pills of unknown origin or a person has been thwacked on the head in a car accident.

If you think about it, our cancer has probably been growing for a long time, and to medical professionals a few more weeks won't hurt that much. While psychologically, we want to GET IT OUT NOW, medically, it's usually less urgent.

So. We must learn how to wait. Here are a few things to know. First, waiting is incredibly difficult for most of us, particularly those of us who are naturally impatient. If waiting in line at the supermarket is painful for you, and the best way to torture you would be to have someone in front of you pay for groceries with nickels and four hundred coupons, then waiting for medical results will drive you nearly out of your skin.

Here's another issue. It's natural to want to change your mood when you feel this sort of anguish. But the things you might typically do to change your mood often don't work when waiting for test results. Exercise, which almost always helps me, was entirely ineffective while we waited to find out about Terry.

Finally, and most important, sometimes we mistake the origin of our internal anguish. Sometimes we recognize that we don't feel right, but start to blame the anguish on the wrong things. Where we live. Our job. Our spouse! Psychologists call this "misattribution."

Remember: While waiting for "big results" you may have negative feelings about everything. Do not act on those feelings. Do not take this out on your spouse, your family, your friends, your coworkers, or your pet fish, Grover. And make good choices about how you are going to change your mood. Do not drink heavily, shop excessively, or imbibe other illicit substances. Do exercise, go for walks, see a movie, talk to friends, and distract yourself. And most of all, remember that waiting is horrible and it is the root cause of your current feelings.

## 2-4. Especially for male caregivers: Don't just do something, sit there.

For most men, their natural instinct is to just figure out what the problem is, fix it, and move on. But no matter how hard you try or how much you plan, you can't fix what's wrong. It's not a broken pipe or a blown gasket, it's cancer.

—Cindy Craddock

It is a helplessness—you want to get in there and fix it, but you can't.

—Bob N.

I think sometimes women underestimate men and their level of ability to care and nurture. We do them a disservice when we do.

—Janice Hallford

If ever there was a time for a husband to become more emotional and just spend more time and listen, this is it. It's a time to man up and be there for your wife.

—Ted Kennedy

The diagnosis of cancer can feel like jet fuel has been poured into our veins. Grab the sword, honey! It's time to rush the field! Charge!

Never mind that the only enemies we have outside our suburban home are garden-invading rabbits and that the cancer is actually sitting quietly in here with us. In fact, when neuroscientists scan the brains of men and women under stress, it appears that men are far more likely to light up the left orbitofrontal cortex, which suggests an activation of the "fight or flight" response. Women, in contrast, light up the limbic system, an area of the brain associated with emotional connection. So there is some research support for a different response to the diagnosis.

For many men, it's painful to not have something obvious to fight. A quick story:

I grew up in an inner-city blighted area of Newark, New Jersey. When I was in second grade, the school population had overrun the aging brick structure, meant for half as many children, and a small gaggle of us were assigned to a large basement closet that had been converted into a classroom. Ms. Pinkney, our elderly teacher, hung cartoonish pictures of famous Americans from the heat pipes, and replaced desks with buckets when hot water sizzled to the ground. She had only a rolling chalkboard as her primary supply, but she wielded an iron hand in the class, using her voice and our first names.

Unfortunately, when class was out, I was left to my own devices and struggled with Rodney, a bully who also had the notable talent of turning his eyelids inside out. The blood-colored underside of his eyelids made him look like some creature that had crawled from beneath the earth to attack me.

Rodney frequently danced up to me when I was on my way home, knocking my lunchbox from my hands or hitting me on the back of my head with rolled-up papers. Our school had recently discovered the mimeograph machine, and "flyers" went home with the students on almost a daily basis.

When I complained to my father one night, seeking and expecting protection, he sat down on the bed next to me and shared that the only way I could escape my torment was to fight back.

*What? Are you insane?* I thought. *Rodney is a killer.* That I hadn't actually ever witnessed Rodney harm anyone didn't enter into my second-grade thinking. In my imagination, Rodney already had a long line of second-grade corpses buried beneath the playground.

Though terrified, I started my campaign by standing up to a friend, Fat Vincent. Vincent weighed twice as much as I did, which wasn't saying much because a cool spring breeze could lift me from the ground, but most of his weight was in his lower half. When Vincent popped me on the head with his hand in anger, I felt that familiar fear, and I tagged him in the cheek with my fist. I think he was more surprised than anything, but he swung back and soon we were both flailing. At some point we got exhausted, and I remember noticing my father standing on the porch watching. I was surprised he hadn't intervened, but then I realized that both of us were crying and finally he said, "All right. That's enough."

Later that summer, I repeated this impressive performance with Rodney, and the two of us eventually became wary friends. (I think we were wary friends because I seemed like a crazy kid who might just suddenly hit someone with no reason.)

Anyway, this lesson was embedded. When afraid, fight. It's much better to have a stinging jaw than tolerate the creeping vulnerability of anxiety. It's a lesson many men have learned.

But, of course, cancer cannot be fought in our playgrounds, sidewalks, or bars. We cannot fix it like a creaking door or rumbling muffler. And as painful as it is, sometimes our central job is to listen to our lovers as they talk about their fears—even as that listening stokes up that horrible anxiety in our bones. This, then, is the real battle. To sit quietly within our skin and with our fears, and listen.

Here's a way to understand the importance of listening from a different perspective. Imagine for a moment that you are in solitary confinement. There's no way out. But every day, someone comes by the cell door and opens the little slit they put food through. Even if they can't get you out, what do you want them to do? Wouldn't you want them to whisper to you that they love you? And listen as you describe what it's like in there? And perhaps tell you that they believe in you, yes?

Let's focus on listening for a moment. I'm going to teach you a specific skill called "validation."

Consider the same conversation from two different perspectives.

*She: "I went in for treatment today and none of the nurses even looked at me. It freaked me out; it felt like maybe something terrible is going to happen and no one's telling me."*

*He: "Those rat bastards. They shouldn't treat you like that. I'm going to go in there and shape them up!"*

In this case, he's responded in the classic "man" approach that whatever she says is a problem that needs fixing. In his mind, he expects her to feel supported and protected. But does she? Probably not. Instead, she likely comes away with the sense that she can't tell him anything. What she really just wants is to be understood. In this specific example, she might have wanted some comfort, too, or the notion that she's probably imagining that the nurses weren't looking at her and even if they weren't, it's probably a reflection of them being busy and not thinking she's about to suffer some horrible fate.

Try this one instead:

*She: "I went in for treatment today and none of the nurses even looked at me. It freaked me out; it felt like maybe something terrible is going to happen and no one's telling me."*

*He: "That sounds scary."*

This is validating. It tells her that he gets where she is and what she's feeling. She's far more likely to say, "Yeah. It was scary."

Or if you want to add some comfort:

*She: "I went in for treatment today and none of the nurses even looked at me. It freaked me out; it felt like maybe something terrible is going to happen and no one's telling me."*

*He: "That sounds scary. Could it be that the nurses were just really busy?"*

*She: "I don't know. Maybe. It was scary though."*

Now let's try a new one:

*She: "My scar hurts. I can barely move my arm."*

*He: "Let's take you into the emergency room."*

*She: "No. It's not that serious. It just hurts."*

Versus:

*She: "My scar hurts. I can barely move my arm."*

*He: "That sounds very uncomfortable. You've been such a trooper lately."*

*(Cue the love scene music.)*

Validation simply states the emotion being expressed.

For men: Our partners often need us to be willing to listen without trying to fix anything. I want you to sit and listen, and tolerate those feelings of anxiety without rushing around trying to do something useful. This takes courage and patience but in the end will be far more helpful, and your partner will feel heard and understood.

When in doubt, validate what your partner is saying by labeling the emotion they express. If you want to offer a "fix" and you just can't help it, offer it in a question instead of a proclamation.

## 2-5. Cancer is expensive. Deal with the financial impact proactively.

It's a nightmare. We're both teachers and make decent money. . . . The hardest thing is the random thing, like, oh, by the way you're going in for a biopsy tomorrow and we need a thousand dollars by tomorrow. That's the thing that's been frustrating, and I've gotten more angry about it. We're not well-off or anything, and a thousand dollars here and there, we don't have that kind of money.

—Tobin Hodges

A recently published study by Maria Pisu at the University of Alabama in Birmingham focused on financial burdens experienced by couples facing breast cancer.[4] She and her colleagues found that during treatment, couples with insurance can expect to pay an additional $300–$1,180 per month on top of their usual spending just for medical costs—and an additional $137–$174 for transportation. These costs decrease but do continue after treatment, with couples paying between $200 and $509 per month in the year after treatment and beyond. While costs will vary by disease, I suspect these estimates apply across the majority of cancers.

In addition, there is a communication gap between physicians and patients. Fewer than 30 percent of physicians ask patients about the how the costs of treatment are impacting them, and similar percentages of patients bring up the costs of medications when it is an issue for them.[5] When patients and physicians do talk about costs, 72 percent of them find it helpful. Physicians can help prioritize medications, find generics when they are available, and learn where the purchase of medications is likely to be less expensive.[6]

The hard part for many couples is that these additional financial burdens come when we are already earning less than before treatment. In some cases, it is possible for both members of the couple to continue working throughout treatment, but in many situations, this is unrealistic—and even if it's possible, many patients need and want their partner with them when they go through challenging treatments.

A research paper published in January 2010 that reviewed more than sixty-four studies showed that between one-quarter and one-half of patients leave their jobs or quit working over the next seventy-two months after a diagnosis. While roughly two-thirds of those will return to work eventually, the majority experience at least some temporary reduction in schedule and wages.[7] By the way, in case you're wondering about long-term issues, when over forty-three hundred long-term cancer survivors were surveyed, only 8.5 percent consider themselves unable to work.[8]

Some people fear losing their jobs if they don't grind through the physical and emotional challenges and continue working. As we will revisit later in a section on privacy and connection, for individuals who work for companies in which there are fifty or more employees, workers have a right to take off twelve weeks (without pay) to care for themselves or a family member. Here's a quote from the United States Department of Labor Web site that describes the law and important details:

*The Family and Medical Leave Act (FMLA) provides an entitlement of up to 12 weeks of job-protected, unpaid leave during any 12-month period to eligible, covered employees for the following reasons: (1) birth and care of the eligible employee's child, or placement for adoption or foster care of a child with the employee; (2) care of an immediate family member (spouse, child, parent) who has a serious health condition; or (3) care of the employee's own serious health condition. It also requires that employee's group health benefits be maintained during the leave.*

In 2009, the president extended and modified these benefits for members of the armed services. More details about these laws can be found on the Department of Labor Web site.

Another available financial tool resides at our insurance companies. Many companies have case managers, often in Human Resources departments, who can be a "one stop" reference point for all of your questions.

But even if we do everything perfectly, bringing every financial tool available to us to bear on the problem, couples still inevitably face a loss. For those of us who have been barely getting by already, this can necessitate painful sacrifices and complex choices. I spoke to couples who could no longer afford to pay for a child's tuition to the school of their choice, or who had to change jobs, and many who quit stressful jobs and either stopped working altogether or took lower-paying, more flexible positions in order to facilitate treatment or recovery.

For individuals who have a great deal of their identity connected to their jobs, these transitions are often painful and come at a time when we are already depleted. For a minority I spoke with, the cancer experience was clarifying—and led patients and spouses to make decisions to leave or change jobs that were more stressful than they were worth, or where office politics were unnecessarily unpleasant.


## 2-6. If there are children in your life, anticipate their concerns and address them.

I am a very active person and when this happened to me they just didn't believe it, really. They just can't think anything bad will ever happen to me.

—Barbara Janzen


A few hours after we learned that Terry had breast cancer I went to the computer and looked up the illness. (See the advice in chapter 1 about not freaking yourself out on the Internet.)

I remember that after I'd looked up the death rates from breast cancer, I closed the search engine and erased the search. I washed my face, calmed my breathing, and walked down the long driveway to meet Alex's bus. I crossed the busy street we lived on and stood waiting for her. Cars passed.

Eventually, her bus pulled up, squeaked, and hissed, the door opened, and our seven-year-old climbed down. She looked at me and then said, "What?" And then again, "What happened?"

Her forehead was lowered and she stared at me like a very short interrogator. "You're a freakish little mind-reader, aren't you?" I said. This did not distract her. From her expression, if she had nuclear eyesight powers, I would have already been vaporized.

"Mom has breast cancer."

"What is that?" She expertly moved her backpack from one shoulder to the other.

"It means she's sick."

"Is she going to have medicine?"

We held hands and crossed the street.

"Yes. It's going to make her tired. And she might throw up." We walked up the driveway, I looked away from Alex into the desert as if I were studying a cactus instead of hiding my face. When I looked back Alex was nodding soberly, like a general who has just learned that her troops have been outflanked.

"Maybe you should make dinner," she said and ran into the house shouting, "Mom . . ."

Here's the thing about kids. They pick up on everything. They are emotional sponges and they study their parents more carefully than we think they do. And even if we don't tell them the whole story, they catch the emotional "vibe" and tend to know when something's wrong, even if we aren't telling them.

So we need to tell them. Because when we don't tell them, they understand something is horribly wrong, but they don't know what it is, and their little imaginations can spark off in all sorts of terrible directions.

Here are the basics:

Kids need the world to be predictable.

Little kids, say seven years and younger, need to know the name of the disease, what the treatment will be like for the parent (in other words, what they might be able to see and hear their parent going through), and as much about scheduling as they can handle. Like if dinner will be different, who's driving them to school or activities, and things like that.

Older kids may want details. How chemotherapy works, why we use radiation, what are the chances that the treatment will work. They may also be called on to assist. In a number of cases, couples with children shared that they had family meetings in which they told their children that the family was going to be different, and everyone needed to pull more of their own weight by doing more chores and work on reducing the stress in the house.

Here's another thing to keep in mind about kids. They often have magical thinking. That is, they believe they can influence things through their behavior or ideas and they may wonder if it's somehow their fault that their parent got cancer. All children have been upset with their parents, so it's critical to tell all children that it's not their fault. Older kids may roll their eyes and say, "Duh" (mine do that occasionally), but it's worth the risk.

When I worked at the Dana-Farber Cancer Institute in Boston I worked with an eleven-year-old boy who was fiercely angry at his nine-year-old brother for causing his mom's cancer. It was an absurd idea, but he thought that if his little brother had been easier to take care of, his mother would not have gotten cancer. It took awhile for us to figure out why he was so angry at his brother all the time, and if we hadn't intervened, we would likely have never known. So generally, now I advocate that every parent say out loud to their children that no one caused the cancer.

The elephant in the room, of course, is mortality. Kids (and we adults) also want to know if the disease will be lethal. Most of the time, we don't know. But in the case of a disease that is likely to be lethal, there are ways to describe this to children when the diagnosis is certain. The gentlest phrase I've heard is, "I'm so sorry, this disease is going to shorten my life."

There is no magic time that makes it the right time to tell a child when a parent is going to die. These are heartbreaking conversations no matter how they are conducted, and having support nearby is critically important. It's also important *not* to try to say things like, "Well, the positive is that you and Aunt Joanie will get a lot closer." There is no positive when a parent dies. And there's no way to truly protect a child from a loss that profound.

More commonly, parents cope with illnesses that present ambiguous threat. With younger children, I see no reason to unnecessarily frighten them, but with older children, the situation is more complex because they may have independent sources of information. Friends of adolescents may know of people who have died of the same illness and may share that information, as in, "Your mom is strong, I bet she does better than my aunt. She died of breast cancer last year."

Adolescents should probably be told that in some situations, these cancers can be lethal, but here are the reasons we are expecting that not to be the case now. This arms them when they get independent information that is threatening from friends or other media.

One complex situation that occasionally arises is when parents disagree over what children should be told about a given situation. I treated a couple who had teenage daughters. The mom was dying of pancreatic cancer and insisted on not telling her daughters the truth. Her husband wanted the children to know, so that they could quit bickering (as adolescents occasionally do) and enjoy the last months they would have with their mother. But mom wanted to live as if things were entirely normal. While understandable, everyone in the household knew that things weren't normal, and this painful insistence on normalcy caused even more anguish. While no rules work in all situations, in these circumstances I generally lean toward truth with older children and adolescents. As much as we try, we cannot protect our offspring from all of cancer's slings and arrows.

## 2-7. Effective couples are flexible about their household jobs and responsibilities during cancer.

. . . like this morning, we've got a dog. I got up and took the dog out. I changed his water and I brushed him, and when David got up he said, "Did you do that?" I said, "Yeah." "Well, why did you do that? That's my job. That's what I do." "OK. Well, you do something else today because I've already done that."

—SANDRA WILKERSON

I am doing a lot of what he did and this aggravates him.

—Barbara Harrison

Just because we have cancer doesn't mean that the laundry doesn't still need to be done, meals need to be fixed, houses need cleaning, and pets need tending. And tires still deflate unexpectedly, water heaters explode, and heavy-footed spouses get speeding tickets (that's a little "shout out" to my wife, who accumulated three tickets in six weeks during chemotherapy, I kid you not).

You have probably split up the jobs in your household. (As an aside, here's some depressing news for us men: Convincing data reveal that couples who share housework do better over the long-term than couples in which only one member—usually the woman—does the vast majority.)

In other areas of your life it's likely that you've managed quite well with only one of you understanding certain realms of your existence. For example, in our household, I do the bills and our taxes and have done them for years. I understand our financial situation. Terry glazes over when I mention accounts and debts and interest rates. It's not that she can't understand, it's just that she's uninterested and her life is incredibly busy and this is one less thing to think about. Similarly, I suffer from child-activity-related dementia and left to my own devices would drive Abby to the airport and Alex to the zoo instead of dance and gymnastics. Unless I'm reminded in the morning, I'm useless. We've come to rely, perhaps too severely, on the other to do what needs to be done.

Then cancer strikes and one of us may be unable to do certain jobs. Or they may be capable, but it may take far more effort for the person who's ill to do that job than it would for the person who isn't ill, or there may be others in the social community willing to pitch in and help out.

Another, more common pattern is that the person with cancer can't do activities on some days but can on others. This is tricky. A number of patients told me that they felt taken for granted or unsupported if they were expected to continue functioning as if nothing was happening when they felt awful, or, at the other end of the spectrum, they felt useless and resented it if their jobs were taken away without being asked.

In my opinion, most couples rely on far too much mind reading. That is, both members expect the other to be able to guess what they need and want, and meet those unspoken needs.

To be effective and flexible, we have to be willing to ask how our partner is feeling and what they are able to do.

1. Remember that having cancer is a new skill. In the past we have been excellent at predicting what we can accomplish in a given amount of time or what we will want to do in the future. But cancer's influence may be unpredictable and the patient may have no way of gauging what she or he will be able to do tomorrow or next week. So both of you will need to be more flexible than in the past.

2. We must forgive our partners for not being able to read our minds or guess what we want without being told. We must both talk about what needs to be done today and who's going to do it.

3. In general, reward one another for talking openly about household tasks. You know, use chocolate, smiles, and touch to let your significant other know that you appreciate them and

their efforts. Say, "Thanks for doing the laundry" and "I appreciate you getting the kids to baseball."

4. Just because you are doing a job today doesn't mean it is yours from now on. I encourage you to continue checking in with one another to assign tasks.

5. Expect some mistakes and rough spots. It's common for the person with cancer to over- or underestimate what they can accomplish. Even regimens that have seemed completely predictable can be suddenly unpredictable.

# 3

# Conquering the Medicine and the Medical Team as a Team

I've worked on two medical television shows, ABC's *Grey's Anatomy* and *Private Practice*. There are many differences between how medicine is portrayed on those shows and reality. First, in real life you may have to give up your firstborn to find a parking spot near a hospital. In real life there won't be four senior physicians standing at your beck and call during all of your treatment. In real life test results don't come back immediately, there are insurance issues, and scheduling surprises. And while everyone at my hospital is as good-looking as they are on those shows, this isn't true of every hospital and clinic. (Oh, and what they call "eternal love" on ABC—when a senior dreamy physician falls in love with a medical resident—in real life we call "sexual harassment.")

Real medicine and medical environments are a very specific culture. To navigate these systems successfully you will need to be prepared to work as a team. From keeping records to communicating with physicians, both of you will play a critical role in order to get everything you need. Of course, there are times in every patient's life when there are minor glitches. There might be late physicians, rescheduled appointments, or confused health-care professionals. Because patients often feel too vulnerable to advocate for themselves, this chapter has a section that teaches partners how to advocate for patients when they feel vulnerable or run down.

Then there's the medicine itself. Behavioral science researchers have shown us that many patients fail to take medications as prescribed, so I've included advice about how to work as a team to improve adherence. Finally, I'll share some information about my experience with unexpected side effects, in hopes that you can avoid the same sort of freak-out that I've experienced and seen many other patients suffer through.

## 3-1. Keep records of everything medical: It will help you avoid quarrels and coordinate care if you need to be seen by more than one doctor.

We started requesting every time we'd go to the doctor, from the urging of another friend that had gone through this, you get every report, you get every scan, you get a copy of everything. . . . There's a few times we'd walk out and go, did they say this or this, did they say that? Then, we'd have that paper to look at and we'd say OK, here's what they said actually. There might not have been a lot of discrepancy, but you got it right there in front of you. Keep up with that.

—David Milson

Navigating complex medical systems can be daunting. Because I've been a speaker to cancer groups for the past ten years (I've spoken in forty-three of our fifty states), I've had a chance to tour every type of cancer hospital and clinic in the country—from massive and famous teaching hospitals to the smallest rural clinics. Some medical systems can be like foreign countries. Just figuring out where to park at a major center can feel harder than putting together a hybrid Toyota from part diagrams narrated in Japanese. And if you have to coordinate care between two or more doctors it can feel impossible.

One of the problems—and this is nationwide—is that we currently lack a unified data bank of patient information accessible by all treaters including doctors, nurses, pharmacists, social workers, and so forth. Instead, our medical system is currently a strange hodgepodge of computer and paper records with no unified standard for information sharing. As a result, unless you have a hand-printed version of your reports to carry with you from physician to physician, you can't guarantee personally that the information will arrive where you'd like.

Consider David and Valree Milson. When David developed lung cancer and thyroid problems and needed cardiac stents, he was treated in Arlington Hospital in Arlington, Texas, Baylor Hospital in Dallas, and the M. D. Anderson Cancer Center in Houston. Valree realized early on that the doctors weren't speaking effectively with one another—and how could they? They were busy, successful physicians who did not have access to the same medical record system. She decided they needed records, so she demanded, after each hospital visit, written copies of every note. While it was occasionally a struggle in the smaller institutions, she was successful in gathering most of the information, and those records made a huge difference when his physicians were confused about which intervention should happen in which order.

In addition, having the records is good for your relationship. David shared with me that sometimes when they left early meetings with physicians they disagreed about what they'd heard. "Having the records helped us understand what we needed to do next and why."

Our capacity to accurately remember information is highly susceptible to stress and anxiety. There were times during my many visits with physicians when my mind was a steel trap, when every word spoken by my physicians or other caregivers was captured. But there were other times—many—when it almost felt like I was underwater, struggling against a current of facts, tests, and the horrible distracting unknown. And sometimes, when we patients meet with physicians, we're literally drugged! We may be halfway through a chemotherapy regimen, preparing to get out of the hospital, or adjusting medications to help us navigate pain or other challenging side effects. Yet people will still try to give us information. I remember clinic visits when I had only recently taken a dose of Ativan, a commonly used drug that evaporated facts faster than water poured into a July desert afternoon. Without someone taking notes, these conversations can't possibly lodge in our heads.

## 3-2. Multiply the surgeon's estimate of your recovery time by three and ask a nurse what's really going to happen.

In the beginning, my husband seemed like a wimp. A total wimp. It kind of disgusted me. Then another patient told me the treatment was harder than the doctor said and I realized he was doing OK.

—Anonymous

Having an inaccurate sense of what the patient's recovery will be like, and how long it will take, often causes problems within couples. If the surgeon says to them, just before the prostate surgery, that he expects the patient to be "up and about in a few days," playfully tapping the man on the shoulder, and then those first days stretch out into two weeks and beyond, his wife may begin to wonder if he's depressed, or maybe there's something wrong? Is he lazy?

At first she badgers him to get up; he's supposed to be fine already. *Is he taking advantage of me while I slave to take care of him and keep the house going?* Meanwhile, he doubts himself and wonders, *Why is she nagging me?*

He may force himself up and about before he's feeling well enough, and risk harming himself. This is a common and potentially serious issue.

Here are two scenarios with the same situation. Imagine that we were going on a raft trip together. And we were headed toward a rapid named "The Widow Maker."

While slowly heading toward the tremendous sound of rushing water, we look over at our guide, who bites at his lip and tells us with a quivering voice to hang on. The boat begins to bounce, we feel the spray in our face, the roar of water squeezing through too small a space; the boat spins and we see the massive rock—a boulder for the ages—approaching.

Now, same situation. But our guide says, "OK, we're headed

toward a rapid they call the Widow Maker. It was named in 1936 when there was a huge hurricane and a foolhardy man went down this rapid in a tiny rowboat and lost his life. That's not happening today. We're going to head downriver, and if you gaze off to the right side of the boat you'll see a beautiful creek joining the river. If you look down, you'll be able to see fifty feet to the bottom and bubbles rising like silver coins. But don't spend too much time looking because I'm going to need everyone to paddle. You're going to feel the boat start to jump and spray in your face. We'll spin around a few times, the boat will press up against the rock, and it may feel as if we are going to capsize but we won't. And then we'll be off and downstream. Ready?"

We all want and deserve surgeons and anesthesiologists who are more like the raft guides in the second category; and believe me, there are those of us in medical education working hard to make sure the next generation of physicians is better than the last. But that won't help you right now. The point is, *We can't expect people who haven't been paying attention to know how to help us make things predictable.*

Surgeons have this problem. When it comes to the smaller concerns of real humans, they have no idea what they're talking about. The formula for recovery uttered by even the most well-intentioned surgeon should usually be multiplied by three. When a surgeon says "You'll feel better in four weeks," this means you will feel better in twelve weeks, and by then you'll want to find the surgeon and scrawl "Liar Liar Pants on Fire" in permanent marker on her lab coat.

As easy as it is to be snarky, I know this isn't their fault. During their lengthy years of training, surgeons spend very little time with recovering patients. They stop by the hospital room the next day and maybe ask for a follow-up visit a month later. They know to worry about pulmonary embolisms—those disks of clotted blood that can weave their way into the fragile lungs—and bleeding, and drops in blood pressure. But they don't know how to make the process of recovery truly predictable for patients.

In the days when home visits were common, surgeons could watch the gradual recovery (or demise) of their patients. But now we don't send them to people's homes. Nor do they do rehab visits, to see what it's like to deal with drains and pains and the fears of walking after cardiac surgery or the way what's happening beneath bandages can frighten us.

Surgeons focus on life at the operating table. This is where they invest their energy. Most of them view time with the patients as an important sideline. Nurses, in contrast, view time with patients as a primary part of their jobs, and most are observant and skilled at managing side effects.

Here's one of the hard parts with getting questions answered. We often don't ask enough questions when we are with physicians. It's intimidating, physicians tend to be rushed, and they often enter the room with a specific agenda. For example, a doctor might enter our room thinking, *Right now I need to make sure Joan knows that she can't eat or drink the night before the surgery.* Or, *In the next few minutes I need to check on Jack's diabetes and make sure it isn't getting worse while we consider our options.* So they enter the room with energy and an approach designed to efficiently get that agenda addressed. But our agenda needs to be "What's going to happen?" and "What's normal?" and "What isn't normal?"

I want you to ask the nurses and other experienced patients, or use reputable Internet resources (hospital-based, for example)—or all of these resources—to find out (1) How long will I (or my spouse) likely be in the hospital after the procedure? (2) How long will I need to stay inactive? (3) What type of side effects from the procedure are dangerous and would indicate that I need to come back to the hospital? (4) I work as a _____; when do you think I should be well enough to return to work? (5) What are the normal challenges after this procedure?

And I want you to be gentle with your spouse if the predicted recovery time is not as expected.

## 3-3. Spouses may need to learn to advocate for their partner.

You gotta trust those people because they have your life in their hands, but you also better protect yourself by making sure that you ask questions. Don't be afraid to ask questions. There's no stupid questions. Ask questions, ask questions.

—DAVID MILSON

I think the spouse can realize they have to step up and be the strong one—the rock—for a while so that the cancer patient can go through what they are going to go through and recover.

—DEBORAH KENNEDY

My biggest advice to anyone today . . . is push, just don't take a doctor's word for something. You just gotta push, push, push. I just didn't take no for an answer.

—LINDA SPENCE

I wouldn't be here if it hadn't been for her.

—HARMAN SPENCE

Let's face it, if we were going to design systems from the ground up to take care of our sickest patients, hospitals and clinics as they currently exist nationwide would probably not come close. While things are improving slowly, we still get our medical care in complex systems that often feel like navigating a rat maze. Teaching hospitals, in particular, offer access to the latest treatments but often leave patients feeling bewildered.

The start of the breast cancer experience is a perfect example. Terry needed to see a breast cancer surgeon, a reconstructive surgeon, an oncologist, a radiation oncologist, and she wanted a second opinion from an oncologist she'd worked with. Oh, and she decided along the way that she wanted a hysterectomy, too— so she needed a gynecological surgeon. And a bunch of anesthesiologists.

Most of those appointments were controlled by administrative assistants. Some of them were kind and organized. Others were terrible. And it felt they had her life in their hands. The same was true of her physicians. A few were brilliant, kind, and dedicated. A few were sloppy and overconfident.

The task of politely getting these people to do what Terry needed occasionally fell to me, especially when she was frustrated and not getting what she needed. Sometimes, I was not polite. I'm not suggesting that we antagonize people unnecessarily, but in medical environments, squeaky wheels do get oiled. Angry family members do get more attention than quiet, polite ones.

Here are a few common situations that may require advocacy by a spouse. Waiting in medical environments is common, but that doesn't mean you should tolerate waits of more than twenty-five to thirty minutes in a clinic without asking for an update. The same goes for waiting to be discharged from the hospital, or waiting for blood counts to be reported by the lab to provide the go-ahead for treatment, or waiting for diagnostic information.

You should have unencumbered access to your medical records so that you can personally make sure all of the doctors you consult have the same information. Ask about access to electronic medical records, sometimes abbreviated as EMR. Some clinics automatically offer notes from each clinic visit immediately, others force us to ask. (We have a legal right to our records, but clinics can make us pay for copying charges.) The same is true for scans, preserved biopsy specimens, and "slides" with our cells on them.

Here's another situation where spouses need to advocate: when the patient is in pain. Pain receives a great deal of bureaucratic attention in clinics and hospitals; hospitals have to prove to accrediting and licensing bodies that they successfully address patients' pain, but that doesn't mean it always happens as quickly as it should. When asking questions about pain, make sure you know which medications your spouse has already taken, and the dosage. Health professionals also routinely ask patients to "rate" our pain on a one-to-ten scale and may also ask us to describe when it started and its quality (burning versus aching versus throbbing).

During a hospitalization, there are many times when spouses may need to advocate for the patient. During the admission process, let intake nurses or nurses' aids know precisely what medications the patient is on, and the dosages. If this is unwieldy, bring the medications to the hospital. Remember that your wireless phone probably has a camera on it—you can take photographs of the pill bottles and show them to the health professionals.

When health professionals bring medications to your room, always ask the name of the med and ask why the patient needs it. While most hospitals are working hard to minimize medication errors, medication errors are the most common mistakes made in acute care environments. There are two types of errors: getting the wrong medication and getting the wrong dosage. While you might not be able to prevent dosage errors, you can vigilantly prevent the wrong medication from being administered.

Spouses can also make sure that no one touches the patient without washing his or her hands first. Infections are the second most common problem in hospitals. There are infections that occur through no one's fault, but there are also infections that are caused by health professionals not washing hands or caring carefully enough for our lines and ports. Most hospital rooms have sinks in them now, where health professionals can "wash in." It can feel intimidating to ask a nurse or physician if they have washed his or her hands, but this is what advocacy is about. It is possible to ask gently, as in, "Doc, I noticed when you came in that you didn't go straight to the sink and wash up. Is that because you aren't going to touch Maggie?"

Don't let a physician's clothing touch your spouse either. No ties, shirtsleeves, jewelry, or lab coats should touch the patient, ever. CBS news *Healthwatch* reported in 2009 that some hospitals in the United Kingdom were banning long sleeves and ties in particular because they are seldom washed and can carry infections from one patient to another.

Another common hospital complaint involves time. Time is experienced differently by physicians and patients. Physicians have busy days, filled with meeting patients, speaking with colleagues, looking up laboratory, pathology, and radiology findings, ordering tests, and prescribing treatments. Patients lie waiting for things to happen. It can often feel as if nothing is happening and sometimes that's true.

For example, it's common for rounding physicians to say something like, "Well, today you can get your catheter out and if you are up and around a bit, we'd like to see you get out tomorrow morning." And then, from the patient's perspective, nothing happens. No one comes to help get the catheter out. Or while approaching discharge, after a mastectomy, for example, the patient needs to be advised how to cope with drains or other medical equipment. But no one appears to explain how they work! In all of these situations, spouses can speak up to nursing staff or other professionals to express the concern.

I suggest starting gently—most health professionals are well intentioned and hard-working—but do escalate if the concern is not addressed. If you are going to complain, here are some things to know. Despite all of the buzz about teamwork, medical systems are still rigidly hierarchical. In fact, if we were anthropologists doing a "medical personnel in the midst" field study, we might classify the rigidity as falling somewhere between an ant colony and the military of feudal Japan. As a result, there is always a supervisor to ask for, and even the CEOs of hospitals (at least the good ones) sometimes personally respond to complaints.

Also, fill out those questionnaires that arrive at your home after a hospitalization. Called "Press-Ganey" after the company that sends them out, or HCAHPS (Hospital Consumer Assessment of Health Care Providers and Systems), these are patient satisfaction questionnaires that are a big deal to institutions who use them to reward and punish clinical units within a treatment center, and, more important, to improve. You'll be doing future patients a service if you are clear about how you were treated.

## 3-4. Work together to improve adherence.

The other day I gave him the wrong medicine . . . and the second I did it I realized it. . . . My granddaughter was here with her friend and I was trying to get a movie for them and get popcorn and he wanted his insulin and it was just too much all at once and I gave him the wrong meds.

—Anonymous

Way back in 200 B.C.E., Hippocrates wrote, "Be alert to the faults of the patients which make them lie about their taking of the medicines prescribed and when things go wrong, refuse to confess that they have not been taking their medicine."

We are now discharging patients who are sick enough that we would have admitted them twenty years ago. That caregivers and patients struggle with adherence is not surprising, given how complex some of our regimens are. For the last six years, in my role as a professor at a medical school, I've been asking medical students to visit patients in their homes and make short video documentaries. One year our students visited a woman with metastatic breast cancer named Norma. A former administrative assistant at a local school system, she was a terrific teacher for the medical students; she let them accompany her to clinic visits and spend quite a bit of time with her at home. One afternoon they were sitting in her kitchen when they asked her how she kept up with all of the medications. Because the interaction was filmed, I can tell you exactly what happened next.

She opened a cabinet and pulled a basket down, setting it on the countertop. She said, "This is everything I have to take." The basket was filled to the brim with medications. They stood, like awkward orange soldiers crammed together in a beach assault vehicle.

One of the students can be heard asking, "How do you keep track of it all?" And Norma says, "I know, huh? Yesterday I forgot to take my Zometa."[1] As it turns out, keeping one's medications in a basket in the kitchen cabinet is not a good way to track medications. And I suspect Norma was doing better than most. In other films, we've seen these baskets in kitchen cabinets, wheelchairs, bathrooms, and bedside tables. This is a common, and terrible, way to track medications.

Unfortunately, studies show that our adherence to recommended medical regimen is generally abysmal. And it's no wonder. In some cases, we need a doctoral degree in engineering to be able to track all of the medications! Some medications need to be refrigerated, others can't be taken with food, others must be taken with food, some need to be taken multiple times per day, others only at bedtime. Some drugs we take only for a specified amount of time, others we take in perpetuity. It's dizzying.

All of us mess up our medications sometimes. At least that's what the research shows. There are actually no conditions for which adherence to medications is even near 100 percent.[2] While we cancer patients can proudly say that we're better at adhering to medication regimen than asthmatics or hypertensives (uh, though some of us have both!), the following are the things that make taking medications less likely:[3]

1. Having to take medications with food
2. Forgetting to anticipate in enough time that we are going to run out of a medication
3. Having to take more than one medication every day
4. Having to take medications multiple times per day

Clearly, there are things we can do to minimize other kinds of mistakes, such as limiting the number of things we are doing at once, not keeping pills that act differently but look similar near one another (that is, don't keep pain medications in the same place as the chemotherapy), and writing instructions down. Like any habit, doing things the same way every day can help us too—most of us are "creatures of habit." The four tricks I've learned from skilled patients for taking medications reliably are

1. Taking medications at the same time every day
2. Using a pillbox
3. Setting up daily reminders (phone or watch alarms work great!)
4. Setting up calendar alarms to remind us to have medications refilled on time

Some of these strategies may feel juvenile. I've heard robust patients say, "I don't need those, I'm sharp as a tack!" But using checklists, pillboxes, and habits to ensure adherence should not be viewed as a "crutch" that only someone with a feeble mind would use. Pilots now routinely use checklists to ready aircraft for flight, medical teams use checklists to ensure safety of patients, and checklists are common in the military.[4] Given that pilots and physicians are typically some of the smartest people in our society, it should be of some comfort that even they need and rely on checklists.

The same year we filmed Norma, we also filmed a young man with AIDS, who also had a complex regimen of antiretrovirals. While he struggled sometimes with other aspects of adherence, he was terrific at taking his pills and he proudly showed our students his large pillbox, which he routinely filled at the start of the month. Using the pillbox and a watch with multiple alarms, he was able to comply perfectly with his medications regimen and did terrifically, successfully improving his CD4 count, a key indicator of health for those with HIV/AIDS.

In addition to the tracking and reminder methods, there are other important factors that influence how often and how successfully we take medications. One is cost. We can ask physicians and nurses about the cost of medications. Unfortunately, two-thirds of patients never talk about the costs of medications with their physicians.[5] When we do, physicians often prescribe less-expensive medications, switch us to generic equivalents, and help us prioritize medications. (Many patients erroneously believe that generic medications are not as good as brand-name medications; we also mistakenly believe that newer medications that cost more are better.) Physicians and nurses will also sometimes know of places where we can purchase medications less expensively. Many patients don't realize that physician groups may purchase infused chemotherapy directly from suppliers, and then sell it to patients using previously negotiated rates. In some cases, physicians can reduce the cost of these medications.

In addition, if we aren't educated about the side effects of specific medications, we are at risk for making mistakes. For example, consider the patient who was on high-dose steroids. Then she started taking a beta-blocker to address some minor cardiac issues. When she next developed stomach pain, she took herself off the most recent medication she'd started, the beta-blocker—but in reality, it was the high-dose steroids that were causing her stomach discomfort, and not the beta-blocker.

Clearly, we should work with our medical teams and not take ourselves off medications on our own—but let's also be honest: many of us do this when we are uncomfortable or have limited access to our treatment teams.

Here's an issue some couples quarrel over related to adherence. All of us have general beliefs about medications. These beliefs may have been passed down from our families or exist in the cultures we come from. I've treated patients who are deeply suspicious of Western conventional medicine and prefer to avoid taking medications no matter what the consequences. I've also treated patients who try to find a medication to match every twitch and twinge.

When individuals in a couple have different fundamental beliefs about medications, this can be a source of friction. The most common fights I've witnessed occur when the patient is in pain and refuses to take pain medications, in an effort to avoid side effects or from a general belief that stoicism and strength are a better match for pain. This sometimes leaves spouses witnessing their loved one struggling with pain helplessly. In some situations, this results in tense arguments in which the spouse feels that the patient isn't helping him- or herself while the patient feels misunderstood and harassed. While there is no simple answer that can address each medication conflict, in some cases, consulting with the medical team can provide solutions that may be unclear to patients. For example, in the pain medication example, taking lower doses of pain medications on a set schedule may ameliorate some of the harsher side effects while providing just enough pain relief to allow the spouse to relax.

## 3-5. Complications don't mean that death is near; almost everyone experiences unexpected side effects. To avoid the mother of all freak-outs, work together to learn and write down the side effects of medications and other treatments.

One consequence of having cancer is that most of us become more vigilant. During my treatments I developed mouth sores, warts, itching, wheezing, shingles, bone pain, gut pain, nausea, nail pitting, and pain with the ingestion of alcohol. I lost the hair on my head, eyelashes, and eyebrows. I peed blue from the dyes from scanners. (Nothing wakes you up in the morning quite as effectively as seeing blue in the bowl—*am I becoming an alien?*) Once, the hair on the right side of my leg stopped growing while the hair on the left side continued to grow. I had every cognitive change imaginable. Once, while septic, I became psychotically paranoid and even hallucinated.

The most challenging of these symptoms occurred deep into my last treatment regimen. I awoke one morning to intense pain in my sternum, specifically my rib cage and the bony plate covering my heart. I knew immediately what it meant: My cancer had metastasized to my bone. (In Hodgkin's disease, once the disease is in the bone there is no chance for cure.) Disheartened, I tried to keep a positive outlook but it was impossible. I decided immediately that I was done with treatment and it was time to go home.

I even rehearsed how I would tell my physician I was done with treatment. I wanted it to be casual-seeming, and dignified, like two well-heeled diplomats discussing the end of a war. If I had a sword, I'd gently hand it over.

My plan was to describe the bone pain and then say, "Well, obviously this means the cancer has spread to my bone, and so I'm ready to return home and stop treatment. Thank you for everything you and the team have done for us. I'm only sorry it didn't work out as we'd initially hoped."

When I met my physician later in the week, I'd gotten so far as to describe the bone pain when he shrugged and said, "Oh, yeah, that's a common side effect of the growth factors we've been giving you." He scribbled in his prescription pad and then looked up, indifferent and a little bored. "Anything else?"

I could barely speak.

When we develop a new, unanticipated side effect, we often wonder if this new symptom is a harbinger of the final curtain closing. *Am I dying?! Is this it?* Most of us can withstand challenging side effects if we know we can alleviate them with other treatments or if they will be temporary.

This frame of mind is especially true of spouses, who are one small step removed from the side effect or symptom. Many spouses suffer quietly, worried that the new side effect is a harbinger of horrible things to come. When both members of a couple get educated about side effects, we stave off unnecessary panic.

Here's an additional problem that's worth understanding. If you read the little inserts (folded up pieces of paper) that come with medications, you'll see that most medications have a long list of possible side effects. There is no way a physician or nurse will tell you all of them; it would take too long, and some patients develop every side effect imaginable if the side effects are suggested to them. It's the opposite of the "placebo effect."

So it's more likely that medical staff will tell you the dangerous side effects or the ones they want you to look out for—as in, "If you develop a fever over one hundred, or a rash, call us."

Because we are not told of every possible side effect, it is inevitable that the patient will develop an unexpected side effect. Unexpected for us patients, that is, not unexpected for the medical staff.

Asking about side effects in advance is a key strategy, and it helps when both members of a couple are present for these conversations. As patients, it is often hard to remember everything we are told (and some of the medications taken frequently may impact our memory directly). To stave off panic when unexpected side effects occur, it is often helpful to have our spouse say, "Hey, don't you remember, Dr. Bob told us you might get X, Y, or Z?"

I strongly recommend not freaking out with every new side effect. Write down what's happening and at your first opportunity ask the nursing staff or your physician the cause. The vast majority of bizarre things that happen in our bodies during treatment have simple explanations.

# 4

# Learn to Deal with the Emotions

Let's face it, the cancer experience stirs up our emotions, and this can interfere with our relationships. Nothing is more disorienting than watching our spouse emotionally spiral out of control. This chapter addresses the most common psychological responses I've seen in couples that cause undue stress.

First, we're going to focus on how to break time into smaller portions to make the challenges more manageable. Then I'll turn to a common coping response many of us use in an effort to protect ourselves—rehearsing bad outcomes. This is largely ineffective and I'll explore why.

We'll cover anger, mood swings, spouse fears, and depression in individual lessons because they call for different strategies. Then we'll turn to a biggie. The most common quarrel I encounter among couples facing cancer concerns optimism. Typically, in this pattern, one member of the couple thinks of him- or herself as optimistic while the other views him- or herself as a "realist." Neither thinks the other is reasonable. I'll trace some of the research that feeds these fights and give specific advice to squelch this painful and needless conflict.

Finally, we'll discuss how we respond to our moods. Our natural tendency is to want to change our moods when we feel down or stirred up. I'll examine some of the choices we often make in these situations and how some of those choices can be destructive. I'll also address the "silent treatment" and how cancer can feed a tendency to not speak about things that bother us because we don't want to "hit the patient when they are down."

## 4-1. After you have a plan, focus on what has to happen today.

We just try to keep busy.

—BARBARA JANZEN

It's easy to get overwhelmed by everything coming. *How will I tolerate sixteen weeks of chemotherapy? What about the surgery? What will hormone therapy do to my body? What about all that radiation? How will I keep the household going and handle radiation treatment? AhhhhhhHH!*

This happens on the spouse side too.

And it's true, if you had to do everything to fight cancer in one day, you'd explode. Fortunately, there's more time. The advantage to having a plan is that you don't have to do it all in one day. Whenever you get overwhelmed by the "big picture," focus on what has to happen today. If that's too much, focus on what you need to do for the next hour or the next ten minutes.

I volunteered in New York State's largest maximum-security prison when I was I college. I worked in a pre-release center, helping inmates prepare for interacting with non-inmates. In reality, I'm not sure I did anything useful, but I did learn quite a bit about prison and, in particular, how inmates coped with challenges.

I was especially surprised that so many of the inmates wore watches. I figured if I were going to spend the better part of my life in prison, I wouldn't want to watch time slowly trickling along. But an older inmate, Ernest Morton, who was ten years into a twenty-five-year sentence for kidnapping, told me I was mistaken. "You can't do your entire bid all at once. You just get through the next little bit of time at a time. Sometimes that's just ten minutes. You time it. And that's how you know you're making progress."

When I had a bone-marrow transplant, this wisdom was enormously helpful. When the intense side effects of transplantation were crashing in, and I couldn't imagine suffering through months of discomfort, I remembered the inmate's wisdom. Breaking up the day into smaller parts was enormously helpful. Instead of worrying about the nausea and weakness I was likely to feel the next day, I focused on today.

When our spouses get caught up and "freak" over the big picture, we can bring them back to now, and what we must do today. We can help them focus on the next little bit of time by asking, "What do you have to do right now?" and "How can we help you be more comfortable right now?" or "What distracting thing can we do together?"

If you are a person who loves to anticipate and prepare for what's coming (like me), this can be difficult. You'd like to know what you need to learn—run out and learn it—and, like a star athlete, be prepared for that situation. But cancer doesn't give you all of your challenges at once. Its challenges unfold at their own pace. We have to be patient and focus on the challenges just in front of us.

## 4-2. Rehearsing bad outcomes doesn't protect us if things do go badly and it usually makes us feel much worse.

Worrying about it never helped anything. I lost a lot of time in my recovery—physically being able to do things that I love to do. While I was still able to do them I should have been enjoying things more instead of worrying.

—Deborah Kennedy

Here's a note to all of you who like to rehearse bad outcomes. (You know who you are.) Do you spend time at stoplights, in the frozen-food section of the supermarket, or in the shower imagining your physician stroking his beard (or hers) or standing awkwardly with her hands in her laboratory coat pockets while telling you that there is irrefutable evidence that you've relapsed, saying, "I'm so sorry the news is not what we'd hoped"? If that's you, then this is for you.

It's natural to want to avoid the experience we had when we were diagnosed—the horrible surprise. The "this isn't really happening" feeling that turns out to be so terribly real. So we rehearse all the bad things that can go wrong in an effort to protect ourselves from being horribly surprised ever again.

But, of course, there are problems with this approach. Many of the horrible things we rehearse don't happen. And while we rehearse, our bodies are listening. Our physiology will respond as if the bad news is real. A distress call is launched in our brains and within seconds, a neuroendocrine cascade of signals leads to adrenal activation, which releases stress hormones like cortisol, endorphins, and epinephrine. A rapid provision of energy is made available through glucose, proteins, fats, and increased oxygen. Our heart rate increases, respiration speeds, pupils dilate, salivary secretions and digestion stop, the bladder relaxes, and we are bolt upright alert, at least for a little while. It's the full fight-or-flight response, which would be ideal if we were about to battle a tiger but isn't so great if you're sitting in traffic, trying to digest lunch, or have just tucked yourself in for a little sleepy-sleepy.

Not only is it physically uncomfortable, bad for our hearts, and bad for our digestion, but here's a hard truth. *It doesn't work.* All the practice in the world doesn't actually prepare us for the horrible feeling of relapsing or learning a treatment hasn't worked. *Nothing can prepare us for that.* There's no rehearsal powerful enough, no way to inoculate ourselves from the terrible disappointment of overwhelming bad news. I tell you this from experience.

So why do it?

The other problem with practicing bad outcomes is that it impacts our relationships. We get snippy with our spouses. Of course, they have no idea that the juice from these bad rehearsals is jetting through our veins. For example, our spouse might be thinking of something normal like dinner, and meanwhile, we're rehearsing the universe exploding. You can see how the dinnertime conversation might be a little awkward or worse. It can also breed resentment. "How can you be thinking about fixing the ice maker while I'm thinking about dying?"

I've also seen and learned of people doing a variety of other unhealthy behaviors while rehearsing bad outcomes in their heads. Overeating, drinking, and my favorite: spending! I had a patient who scoured Internet shopping sites while her mind went to dark places. It resulted in some odd and expensive purchases.

Stopping the rehearsals takes practice and focus. We tend to be in a trance-like state, only half aware even that we're doing it at first. It can be helpful to share with our spouse that we're having darker thoughts and ask for help distracting ourselves. Engaging movies, exercise, and activities with other people can help.

Patients have also shared with me that with practice, we can stop the rehearsals by first recognizing that they are happening and then acting to distract ourselves or by rehearsing more positive outcomes.

The reality is, we usually don't know what the future holds. But wasting our time now painting it black can ruin our present.

## 4-3. We patients can be moody and unpredictable. Muzzle anger.

One time in particular I remember, it was on a Friday evening while I was in treatment, and I mentioned something about trying to get up on Saturday morning and go to the gym. A. J. asked me if I really thought that was a good idea. I became so angry with him for questioning me. Did he think I wasn't well enough to work out? And who was he to question me about my decisions as he was not a doctor?

My anger then escalated as I started thinking about how he had not gone to my doctor's appointments with me, and if he had, he would have known that my doctor said it was fine to exercise. Anyway, Saturday morning rolled around and I did not feel well enough to work out. When he asked me if I was going to the gym, I became so upset that he was insensitive to me and my illness and that he really did not realize how sick I was. The whole two-day exchange was a complete contradiction where neither one of us (especially me) did a very good job of communicating with the other.

—Elissa Bantug

We all get chemo PMS.

—Tyson Rudd

Here's a pattern I've seen frequently.

Sometimes when we feel robbed, we lash out at our lovers. This often makes sense. In the past, they've often been guilty as charged! When I come home after a long day and someone has thrown out the soup I was saving, chances are, it was Terry. When there's less in our checking account than I expected, it's her. And when the floor is covered with the work slacks and work shirt that I have forgotten to pick up (and tie and shoes and . . .), it was me. Guilty, your honor.

But when cancer robs us, sometimes we behave the same way, as if our spouse has imbibed all of our cosmic soup, left the shirt on the floor, and emptied the bank account all at once.

Many of the patients I spoke with mentioned how angry they occasionally became at their spouse, often for crimes that, prior to the diagnosis, would have been met with only a playful grimace.

There are a flood of biological changes that can induce fierce anger and sadness. Screeching into menopause, coming off of steroids, intense fatigue, pain, and general discomfort can all intensify these feelings.

A special word about anger: When we express fear and other emotions, we usually feel better. But not anger. Anger, like fire, feeds on oxygen. Expressing it often stokes, rather than depletes, the anger. It's worth remembering, in these moments, that our spouses are stumbling through this, too. That this is hard on everyone that cancer touches.

Even when we are well intentioned and think we have a handle on an issue, we often give more energy to what we're saying than it deserves. When I was sick, I remember fighting with Terry about my tendency to park far away from the grocery doors. She had only remarked that there were closer spots, but I launched into a tirade and then was surprised at the vehemence in my language, the tone I'd assumed. Overhearing us, you would have thought she'd threatened to beat our children.

(Some readers, particularly those who NEVER express anger and prefer silence, are feeling a little smug just now. Don't worry, oh, you masters of the silent treatment, we'll get to you soon.)

Here's my advice: Angry feelings have a beginning, a middle, and an end. Given enough time, they end. Turn down the volume, the intensity, and the fire. And if necessary, clamp down on anger until the feelings pass. They will. They do. Do not take your anger out on your spouse or family. Cancer is not their fault. It is happening to them, too. I'm not suggesting that we stop discussing important issues, only that we make an exhaustive effort to do so when we feel our calmest.

There are reasons to calm our anger. It appears that arguments with our spouses do have a direct impact on our health. A couple of researchers (who are also a married couple) at Ohio State have been researching the impact of arguing with our spouses on our health. Ronald Glaser, an immunologist, teamed up with his wife, Janice Kiecolt-Glaser, a psychologist, to study marital fighting. In one experiment, they invited a couple into the lab. They used a suction cup to blister one of their arms repeatedly. (Yes, they paid them handsomely.) Then they asked the couple to have a supportive conversation. On another day, the couple repeated the blistering but were asked to have a conversation about a topic they frequently fought about.

The results were impressive. On days when the couples argued, the blisters took a full day longer to heal. When the couples were especially hostile, the wounds took two days longer to heal![1] In fact, they noted that couples who showed greater hostility in general healed at only 60 percent of the rate of couples who argued with less hostility.

Another study was conducted by a friend of mine, a neuroscientist and psychologist from the University of Virginia. Jim Coan recruited women who were happily married to be in a study in which they allowed their brain to be scanned while they were threatened with shock. Some of the women held hands with a stranger, some of them held their lover's hands. When they were holding their lover's hand, they showed the same soothing response in the right anterior insula, superior frontal gyrus, and hypothalamus that we typically see when patients take opiates (strong pain relievers). In fact, the stronger the marriage, the less threat the brain seemed to perceive from the shock.[2]

So take it down a notch. Soothe the anger. Hold hands against the threats.

## 4-4. Cancer treatments and fear can induce wild mood swings. It's a good idea for caregivers not to take these personally.

Once in a while she would cry and I would think it was me until we talked matters over and I knew what was what. My initial reaction sometimes was "What did I do wrong now?" or whatever.

—RAY LABONTE

We have had times when each one of us will get really upset and yell. She just lets it out when it happens.

—RICHARD KELLEY

The cancer experience is rife with mood swings for many of us. Cancer makes us scared, and then we respond to vulnerability with all sorts of emotions. We can be irritable, anxious, angry, sad, or any combination of these. For many of us, trying *not* to think about cancer can also be like a magnifying glass that blows normal emotions up and amplifies life's little insults.

Many of the patients I spoke with noted that their emotions exploded when something simple in their life happened. Barbara Janzen told me a story that happened one month after she was diagnosed. She was going out to a party and before she left, she hid her purse in the washing machine because a family member had warned her family that they could get robbed. This is how she described what happened next.

> Then my husband brought me home and he said, "I'm running out of underwear," so I went and threw underwear in the washer and put in the bleach and let the washing machine run. Then my washing machine was flying all over the place, it was in the middle of the floor. . . . I opened it up and there was my pocket book. The strap had gone over the ringer and everything was, well, you could imagine. I just slammed the lid down. And that is when I cried—I guess about my cancer. I just stood there and cried and cried.

Some cancers also directly cause mood swings by deregulating hormones or impacting neurotransmitters, those little messengers that run between major brain structures. Cancer treatment can also be a mood killer. Removal of a cancerous thyroid, for example, can induce hypothyroidism, which, in turn, can induce sluggishness and depression. Anti-estrogen drugs used to combat estrogen-positive breast cancer can also cause the onset of menopause and a deregulation of emotion.

Barbara Andersen, a psychologist and researcher at Ohio State who focuses on cancer, has shown that the cancer experience often impacts cortisol, epinephrine, norepinephrine, and ACTH (these are hormones that help us prepare for stress) and that these are directly tied to our experience of pain, fatigue, and depression.[3] In other words, our bodies and minds are part of the same system, and an assault on one part biologically impacts the other parts.

Many chemotherapy agents can also impact mood. Prednisone, which oncologists use frequently, can cause terrible anxiety and depression when we stop taking it, as our adrenals struggle to catch up.

Of course, we had lives prior to developing cancer. A major risk factor for mood problems during cancer is a history of depression or anxiety prior to the cancer diagnosis.

Couples who have been close for years are typically good at reading one another's moods, and it's common for us to blame those closest to us when we feel upset. It's also normal for spouses to wonder why a partner is upset at them. Some of the men I spoke with noted that when their spouses were sad or angry or irritable they frequently wondered what they had done to upset their significant other. They also sometimes felt responsible for fixing the problem, whatever it might be. Unfortunately, this usually made things worse, as the patient felt distanced from the spouse.

Bob N. told me a story about taking his wife, a patient, on a beautiful scenic autumn drive to distract her from everything happening. He shared,

> It was perfect. And we get back to our house and she is in the kitchen and all of a sudden she is breaking down, bawling. And I say, "What's wrong? We had a great day" and I thought we kept her mind off all of this. Of course, I'm not keeping her mind off it, she is thinking about it the whole time. And then she said, "It was such a gorgeous day; it was so beautiful. It was just so pretty up there, and the perfect time of year, and I'm just wondering if this is the last fall I'll be able to do that."

He told me he was devastated. Though he knew later it wasn't really his fault, in the moment he blamed himself for putting these thoughts in her mind.

This is how I explain it to spouses in couples' therapy when

I've seen this pattern. Imagine for a moment that you are in a tiny lifeboat, alone, and a school of huge sharks is swimming all around, with those indifferent, lifeless eyes and rows of big teeth. You're terrified. Your spouse is on the phone and asks, "Why are you being so angry all the time, what did I do wrong?"

We cancer patients carry those sharks around in our heads. They come with us to the supermarket and on beautiful scenic drives, and it isn't the spouse's fault the sharks are there. And we do want to be distracted, but there's only so much distraction that's realistically possible. And sometimes we're going to be angry and sad and confused, and those feelings aren't the spouse's fault either. They just are.

## 4-5. For lovers: Saying, "I'm scared too" out loud will not rip a hole in the universe, and it might bring you closer. But if you say it too much, it will bum everyone out.

I think many [people] are scared to express how they feel or put their feelings out there as they view this as being selfish while their wife or husband is battling something so scary as cancer. I wish he could have spoken to me about his fears of me dying, not being able to have children, etc.

—Elissa Bantug

One minute he fell out in the backyard and he just laid out there and cried and you just don't expect to see your husband in that condition.

—Barbara Janzen

Terry and I are in the car. The kids are asleep in the backseat. We've just sought relief from the desert summer at a water park in Phoenix. She felt well enough to go, and I think we were both eager to feel normal . . . whatever that is. Chemotherapy is coming, but she's been given four weeks between her surgery and the start of chemo to recover.

On the way up we argued about the ecological disaster that is a water park in the middle of the desert—with its rapidly evaporating wave pool and lazy river, slides, and squirting frogs, rabbits, and trees. But we went ahead and widened our carbon footprint anyway, by driving the kids up Route 10 to Phoenix, and now, on the way back, everyone is sun-kissed and sleepy.

"You've been quiet," Terry observes looking out her window. "What are you thinking about?" she asks. I hesitate, just a second too long.

"Nothing."

"Nothing?"

"I heard my department's getting hit with new cuts," I offer.

"Oh," she says. "Bummer. Who will it impact?"

"The clinicians," I say.

"Hmmmm," she says.

It seems innocuous enough, but she's too perceptive for me. She knows I'm thinking about something else and even as she looks out the window there's disappointment in her voice.

"That's what you were thinking about?"

"Uh."

*NO!* I want to scream. *Of course not.*

After Terry's breast cancer diagnosis, I didn't know how much to tell her. I'd always just told her what was on my mind and in my heart. But now, when my mind was haunted by what might be, this seemed uniquely inappropriate. When she wasn't around, or when I was watching a movie or show that was supposed to be emotional—like the death scene in *Steel Magnolias*, or even child movies like *Spy Kids*, which the kids think is all about fancy-technology-flying kids saving the universe but is actually about families and love and intimacy and having a mother and father—I'd cry nearly uncontrollably in the dark. But with her, I stopped telling her what I really felt.

The research literature confirmed that I was not alone in this approach. A careful team of behavioral researchers at the Seattle Cancer Care Alliance—a talented group who worked at the University of Washington, the Fred Hutchison Cancer Center, and Seattle Children's Hospital—compared caregivers' language and nonverbal expressiveness when alone versus when their spouses were present. They discovered that when they were alone, spouses of cancer patients frequently spoke openly about the challenges of cancer and that their nonverbal descriptions were negative and consistent with the content of what they were saying. But when the spouse was around, they were positive, even when they felt bad and afraid. In other words, they routinely hid their real emotions.[4]

This is entirely understandable. What kind of spouse wants to be a downer? But at the same time, this falseness can drive a wedge. How much can we be "in this together" if one of us is pretending that things are fine and "looking up" no matter what the evidence on the ground?

Of course, there's minor secrecy in all relationships. And routine ways we lie to our spouses. The "No, you look great, let's go" when the babysitter has finally arrived and we're late to meet friends for dinner but my wife is wearing a dress that was cut specifically to make her slender waist appear as if she'd swallowed a goat. Or "I'm OK with how much you spent on that coat even though you have another one that looks remarkably similar and you never wear that one either even though it fits and you look great in it." And perhaps deeper ways. The ways in which we don't match one another that we keep to ourselves.

But her cancer experience felt a little like the beginning of the roller coaster when we're going up the severe incline, one of us trembling and one of us—well, me—pretending to be thinking about budgetary issues at work.

Instead of sharing my experience, I frequently went quiet. We'd be on our way somewhere and she'd say, "You're quiet," and I wouldn't say that I was worried about her blood counts or that the muscles around her implants were going to retract with the radiation or that it would just be me and these two little girls and instead I'd just say nothing. Or I'd make something up that she'd be interested in like a meal we might try to make or a college football game or a show she'd probably like, but she'd respond softly, as if she'd caught me, uninterested in my distracting subterfuge, and on some level wondering about what was in my heart.

As a result of my growing expertise at quieting, she sometimes thought that I wasn't thinking about breast cancer at all. That I took for granted how well she coped, how strong she was, and she'd incorporate some breast cancer comments into a conversation like, "Well, I didn't get to the laundry because of the whole surgical recovery thing, not that you've been thinking about it much," even though those surgeries and the coming chemotherapy were so bright that it was like an airport searchlight that blazed into my eyes and I couldn't think about other things. And I couldn't shoot back, "Well, yeah, I'm thinking about the cancer, it's all I *do* think about" because that would make her feel worse.

And maybe also I was afraid that if I opened that box in front of her, so much would tumble out that I'd be nonfunctional, eager for sleep, and unable to work. I even started collecting amusing anecdotes so that if pressed, I'd be armed with something to say. Anything other than that the universe was listing dangerously to the left and I've scratched my fingers raw looking for the life jackets.

I heard conflicting advice about this topic from couples on the front line, and I think that's because the truth is a complex mixture of both for most of us. On one side, a minority of patients want their lovers to be normal, and happy, and even avoid bringing up all challenging topics. Some patients I spoke with, especially women, complimented their men on being "like a rock."

Others long for greater intimacy, truth, and authenticity. They want their lovers to acknowledge their own fears, and not shield them from the normal slings and arrows of daily living.

Having been both the spouse and the patient, here's my advice: When I was ill, I wanted to know that the people around me cared enough to worry about what was going to happen. Unfortunately, when we're sick and feel vulnerable, it's easy to mistake a lover's stoic response for a lack of caring. We want to know that they love us so much that they're scared.

Meanwhile, on the other side, the patient needs to know that we are now—and will be—functional. When Terry became ill I learned that she needed me to look strong and capable. She knew

I was terrified, but she wanted to be confident that no matter what happened, I'd be able to help her and keep our household going.

So for us it was a subtle dance between these two poles. On the one hand, it was important that I tell Terry how scared I was. On the other, I had to look strong. The reality is, we can do both. Even simultaneously. And acknowledging our fears of what might happen doesn't actually make those things happen. And it can bring us closer.

I want you to find that happy medium that balances authenticity and honesty with sucking it up and not being a tremendous downer.

## 4-6. If either of you develops depression, get it treated!

I was terribly depressed for the first part of June and my wife said something to the doctor. That's the furthest from who I really am. My dad had depression and was manic-depressive. So I had witnessed some of that stuff as a kid growing up. I said that will never happen to me. I'm telling you, you don't have any control over it. It comes. It blindsided me. It's been a struggle.

—DAVID MILSON

Everyone has challenging times during the cancer experience. But prolonged periods of absolute darkness define depression, which can be relieved, frequently, with treatment.

Depression is common among patients—with a mean-point prevalence of between 15 percent and 30 percent[5] at any given time (this is as much as five times higher than the rates in the general population). And—here's the part you may not realize—it is equally as common in the spouses of patients as it is in the patients themselves.

In addition, partners are far less likely to be diagnosed or seek treatment—with one study showing that patients received treatment for their depression 58 percent of the time, while partners only received treatment 34 percent of the time. That's right, only one-third of partners ever get help.[6]

Let's back up for a second. There are a number of reasons why partners don't get help. In general, many partners stop taking care of themselves physically. They may say to themselves, "I need to focus on him right now." And, "Of course I feel down; anyone would." While these statements are partially true, they are also excuses for not getting help. And in the swirl of extra tasks—picking up prescriptions, keeping food on the table, and meeting work obligations—self-care can fall in priority.

In my field we frequently remind patients and partners of the words we hear from flight attendants for mothers sitting next to children: "If oxygen masks should descend from the ceiling, put your mask on first, and then put the mask on the person sitting next to you."

If you or your partner is depressed, I strongly advise you to get help. Therapy (individual, group, couples, and family), medications, acupuncture, exercise, light boxes, and combinations of these have all been shown to effectively relieve depression when done well. Other, less proven but potentially successful, treatments for depression include herbal supplements, massage, yoga, and dietary changes. I also have a friend named Robert who has cured his depression by leaping into freezing water, but I don't recommend it. Except for him. Robert looks funny when he shivers.

## 4-7. Stop fighting over how your partner is thinking about cancer.

I kept telling her, trying to be positive, maybe your hair will just thin out, maybe you won't completely lose it, and she doesn't like that, she doesn't want to hear that. I don't know what she wants but she doesn't want to hear the best-case scenario from me.

—Tobin Hodges

I would hear, "It's not that bad," and David would hear, "Yeah it's that bad."

—Valree Milson

He was focused on "you probably don't have cancer" instead of "even if you do have it—it will be fine." . . . It felt like unrealistic optimism and he turned out to be wrong.

—Deborah Kennedy

Consider Tobin Hodges, a young man with a one-year-old child and a young wife recently diagnosed with stage 3 Hodgkin's disease. Her hair is trickling out. Tobin wants his wife to think positively, but she wants to prepare for being bald.

The most frequent argument I hear between couples in which one or both members have cancer concerns thinking and attitude. I heard some common statements during my work and interviews with patients and spouses:

"He's such a cheerleader."

"She's so pessimistic all the time."

"I like being prepared for the worst; she wants me to be positive."

"He's killing himself with his negativity."

"I wish she would stop seeing everything as half-full."

Here's the crux of the argument: The patient wants to prepare for the worst and not get blindsided by any more horrible surprises. But the caregiver believes that through positive thinking, the patient might keep his or her energy up and perhaps even destroy the cancer with a positive attitude.

These are incompatible beliefs: In order for the patient to get what he or she wants, the worst-case scenario must be considered and planned for. In order for the caregiver to get what he or she wants, the worst-case scenario should never be considered and especially not discussed. The patient may also want to hear from his or her partner that even if some bad stuff happens, we'll get through it. We can handle it. The caregiver's refusal to contemplate these negative outcomes can leave the patient feeling vulnerable. *Will she be able to handle it if things don't go like she's thinking they will?*

In Tobin's case, he compromised. He shared, "I had to listen to what she was saying and instead of saying 'Maybe her hair will stay in,' just tell her that 'It doesn't matter, if this is the worst thing we have to deal with in this situation then we're pretty blessed.'"

A few of the couples I interviewed had quarreled from the very start, even before the cancer was diagnosed, and this early argument had cast a shadow over subsequent treatment. In those cases, the partner had tried to encourage his spouse by telling her he didn't think "it" would be cancer, but then, indeed, "it" was cancer.

The principle here is that the patient wants to feel that the most likely scenario in the near future can be tolerated. In my opinion, having played both roles, there's a balance here. The patient can be allowed to briefly discuss realistic possibilities in order to feel prepared, but when they spiral into catastrophizing, it's a good time for the spouse to speak up. The exception is when the patient is depressed and rejects any optimistic idea out of hand.

To explain why these fights occur with such frequency, let's take a very quick trip through research and pop culture, starting in the late 1960s. I'm going to share some scientific research with you, but hang with me, I think you'll find it's worth the effort to understand this.

In 1968, Martin Seligman and his colleagues published a study of dogs and conditioning. In his seminal study, Seligman and his colleagues had three groups of dogs. The first group was put into a hammock that they could not escape from and then they were shocked for eighty-five seconds (I know, who thinks of these studies?!). Typically, these dogs howled for a while and then passively accepted their fate.

A second group was put into a hammock that was escapable and then they were shocked. Typically, dogs in that condition wriggled once the shock started and successfully escaped the hammocks.

A third group received no shock. Then Seligman and his colleagues put all three groups of dogs into a new shock-giving "shuttle box." For all of the dogs the shock was escapable. The box had two sides. On one side, there was an electrified grid on the floor. On the other side of the box, beyond a small partition that the dogs could easily jump, there was a nonelectrified floor. A buzzer went off, warning the dogs that shock was coming.

Here's the thing. In the shuttle box, shock was escapable. The dogs could easily jump over the little fence once the warning sounded, and escape the shock.

Dogs who had been in the escapable hammock usually figured out that the other side of the box was safe and quickly learned to avoid the shock. Dogs who hadn't been in a hammock at all also escaped quickly. But dogs that had received inescapable shock while in the hammock rarely escaped the shock in the shuttle box. And check this out—those same helpless dogs occasionally wandered over to the other side of the shuttle box (which was safe) when the buzzer went off—but they still didn't learn that the shock was escapable, and in future trials they just quietly yelped and suffered when the shock buzzer sounded.

Seligman and his colleagues realized that the dogs in the inescapable hammock had learned that they were helpless to impact their environment. The dogs hadn't realized that the helplessness was limited only to the hammock—that when they were in the shuttle box, they could escape. They coined the term "learned helplessness" to describe this phenomenon.[7]

The next natural question was, did this apply to humans? As it turned out, absolutely. Using noise, cognitive problems, and other stressors, researchers have repeatedly demonstrated that humans behave just like the dogs.[8] If we learn that we are helpless to impact our environments in an important way, it often generalizes to many other situations. There's also evidence that there are neurological correlates of helplessness—rats, for example, show depletion of norephinephrine, an important neurotransmitter for mood—when they have been conditioned to learned helplessness.

Further research has shown that helpless thinking causes, and is a symptom of, major depression. In other words, we can think our way into depression. Cognitive behavioral psychologists have revealed that it is also possible to think our ways out of depression by challenging some of our helpless beliefs.[9]

When I was in graduate school in the late 1980s, a group of researchers tried to take a leap with this research. They believed that helpless thinking, in contrast to a "fighting spirit," would result in different levels of mortality in cancer patients. That is, they felt that patients might die sooner if they had that same helpless or negative—what the researchers called "resigned"—thinking.

Around the same time Bernie Siegel published his book *Love, Medicine, and Miracles* (1986), and these ideas shot through the popular culture. Many people believed that in *Love, Medicine, and Miracles,* Siegel, a surgeon, was arguing that with correct, optimistic thinking, determination, and self-love, people could miraculously cure their cancers. In reality, Siegel was probably doing two things at once. He was allowing the publicity around his book to be driven by the promise of miracles, while simultaneously his real message was subtler—that self-love and determination are important for all humans and a rare, occasional result might be a miraculous outcome.

But this subtlety was lost on the general population, and to his enrichment.

An unfortunate by-product of Siegel's thinking was "New Age

guilt." This is the idea that if you develop cancer, if you relapse, or if you aren't quickly cured, you must be thinking incorrectly, negatively, or without enough self-love. New Age guilt was stoked again in this culture when the 2006 self-help book *The Secret* shot up best-seller lists. Like Siegel's writings, *The Secret* promoted the idea that using correct thinking brings positive physical results. While neither book says this directly, a common conclusion drawn by patients is that if we become sick, or relapse, or otherwise struggle with our health, we must be thinking "wrong."

But let's step back and think about this. Is this true?

Let's consider a few examples of amazing thinkers. One need only consider the incredibly brave, wise, optimistic, and determined Christoper Reeve (aka Superman) or Randy Pausch (of the famous "Last Lecture") or Morrie Schwartz (from Mitch Albom's *Tuesdays with Morrie*) to see that the connection between thinking and health outcome is not clear. These three men were remarkable—and there are countless more.

Here's the other truth. Everyone—I mean everyone—has down days when they have cancer. It is absurd to blame ourselves or our spouses for feeling down, or weary, or even angry. We already have a heaping plate of cancer. Most of us don't need an extra helping of guilt.

So how should a supportive spouse respond when we are waiting for test results? What should they say? In these situations I strongly advise couples use "survivor optimism." We're strong together and we can cope with whatever comes our way. And let's all ease up on blame. There is no conclusive evidence that thinking positively or negatively results in greater mortality from cancer.

## 4-8. It's adaptive to want to change our mood when we feel down; we just have to be careful about what we choose.

From the days of spinning ourselves around on playground equipment to climbing trees or holding our breath—it's a natural part of the human experience to want to change our perspective.

And when we're down, it's natural and adaptive to want to do something to change our mood. Often, the things we choose are healthy. We may pour ourselves a glass of wine, take a bath, call a friend. We can go for a walk, read an engaging story, write a blog, or take a nap. And there's more! We can exercise, go for a drive, meditate, eat chocolate, watch a movie, or even—*gasp*—some strange people like to clean things. No kidding, like actually cleaning out the garage makes them feel better.

But some of our choices are less adaptive. Some behaviors effectively change our mood in the short term but are risky for us or our relationships over the longer term. Some of those risks are social—we may alienate the people closest to us—and some are physical—we may harm or put ourselves at risk. Other risks are financial or even threaten our jobs or freedom.

Before I explain a few of these further, let me just remind us of Grandma's wisdom about moderation. Most of these behaviors are fine in small amounts. It's kind of like how we view medication. The only difference, in many cases, between a medication and a poison is dose. A little of any of these things is usually OK. But too much and we put ourselves and often our loved ones and our relationships at risk.

And let's not underestimate how much anguish comes packaged with the cancer experience. It can be an electric juice that fires us up and leaves us few outlets for feeling better. It is no wonder some of us choose behaviors that are sometimes troubling.

## Spending

I've known patients who have gone on prolonged spending binges—purchasing exotic items on eBay or in shoe stores, for example. I've known patients or family members who have purchased cars, clothing, furniture, jewelry, and even houses.

As I mentioned earlier, one person I treated went online and made thousands of dollars worth of eBay purchases of household items she'd always admired. Then she tried to hide the purchases—which resulted in fierce battles with her husband, who was shocked when he discovered the thousands of dollars in expenditures.

She loved the hunt for objects—the careful searching, inspecting, and researching—and this was a mostly healthy distraction. But she was also on high doses of narcotics for pain, and other drugs that influenced her cognition, and she occasionally bid on, and won, unintended objects—including some that were extremely large. Her spending was destructive because it threatened her relationships.

Some of my patients had a long history of using consumer therapy when they felt down. A trip to the mall or boutique was just the thing they needed when the world's harshness took on too sharp an edge. A new pair of shoes or a handbag could ameliorate weeks of anguish in a flash. But when the challenge is too large—like cancer—the shopping therapy can lose its power to quench the anguish, and some patients spend more and more, chasing that elusive elixir of calm that once flowed so easily.

Let's face it directly: When cancer is the problem, new objects are rarely the solution.

## Eating

Isn't food wonderful?

Some of us are accustomed to looking to food to improve our mood. Food can be fantastically social, stimulating, and satisfying. And for those of us whose are routinely experiencing unpleasant side effects and symptoms, or feel that our physical selves have betrayed us, food can be one of the few activities that still bring us physical pleasure.

Unfortunately, for many patients, the cancer experience is also associated with weight gain. While some patients suffer significant appetite suppression with cancer, many others gain significant weight. Part of the weight gain may be related to changes in metabolism, and some of it may be related to medications that induce increased appetite, such as steroids. But weight gain is also often a product of confusing anguish for hunger, and trying to change one's mood through eating.

Rapid weight gain can interfere with relationships. It can render previously enjoyed physical activities too hard to accomplish, increase fatigue, and induce self-loathing that in turn eclipses sexual desire and closeness.

In addition, there is growing data that obesity is associated with increased rates of relapse. I'm going to cover food and diet in a later chapter in more detail. For now, if you are one of those folks who sometimes confuses anxiety and hunger, it's worth considering doing something to specifically address anxiety (exercise, distraction, meditation, yoga, talking with friends, writing) before eating.

Like most biological longings, we can wait out our urges to eat. Putting some time between the first urge to eat and consumption can reduce the calories we consume. When we do eat, we can also be more selective about the calories.

## Alcohol

In the words of one alcoholic I treated, "I drink alcohol because it works. It makes me feel better. At least for a little while." Alcohol is readily available, socially acceptable, and it effectively changes people's moods.

As many as 30 percent of adults in the United States report having some form of alcohol use problem at some point in their lives. Interviews with nearly fifty thousand adults also revealed that fewer than one-quarter of these folks ever sought or received help.[10] The lead author of this massive study, Deborah Hasin at Columbia University in New York, concluded that high alcohol usage is one of the most disabling and prevalent disorders in the country.

Biologically, high alcohol intake deregulates natural circadian rhythms. It interrupts sleep and eating patterns, leading drinkers to go to sleep too late or too early, and high alcohol users often don't eat during the day and then binge at night. This can lead to a cycle of drinking to fall asleep and still not getting decent rest, which results in greater vulnerability to stress, irritability, and . . . you guessed it, more alcohol usage.

I've seen more problems with alcohol (in patients and family members who had no problem with it before) than any other behavior. In my field, we are somewhat equivocal about alcohol. "Well . . . ," my colleagues sometimes say, "if it isn't harming your ability to work or your relationships, it isn't a problem." And this is reflected in our diagnostic system. In order for a patient to be classified as abusing or being dependent on alcohol, it must interrupt key social functions or cause the drinker significant distress. But this is often difficult to gauge or define and, honestly, many people are good at juggling high alcohol intake and the superficial aspects of their jobs and relationships. And when cancer strikes, they blame any diminished function on the cancer—not the alcohol.

Here's the criteria I want you to use: If you are drinking more than two drinks per night, or drinking in places or situations in which it's prohibited (like driving or sneaking it into the hospital—*I kid you not*), then it's a problem.

There is a great scientific effort under way right now to understand the relationship between alcohol intake and cancer risk. Occasionally we will see new publications that announce that alcohol—usually red wine—in moderate amounts reduces cancer risk, but most of the research points in the opposite direction. High alcohol intake has been linked to increases in breast, colon, prostate, and head and neck cancers.

Newer research is focusing on those of us who have already had cancer. A recent study of breast cancer survivors revealed that consuming three or more drinks per week was related to a 1.3-fold increase in risk of recurrence. Marilyn Kwan and her colleagues followed almost nineteen hundred women and found that especially among women who were overweight or obese, alcohol consumption beyond three drinks per week was related to increased recurrence.[11]

There's some laboratory work to explain why. Researchers at Rush University Medical Center showed that alcohol can make cancer cells more aggressive, and that it particularly impacts the epithelial-to-mesenchymal transition, which plays a key role in metastasis—the spread of cancer cells.[12] Other researchers have studied telomere lengths, which are proxies for our biological age. Found at the end of chromosomes, telomeres are important for the genetic stability of cells, and shortened telomere length is related to increases in cancer occurrence. Heavy alcohol use resulted in dramatically shortened telomere length, presumably through oxidative stress and inflammation.

In addition to the increases to physical risk, alcohol usage also threatens relationships. Some of us are quicker to anger when inebriated. Others are withdrawn, forgetful, or prone to emotional swings. Few are viewed as reliable, steady, or, most important, connected. Here's the bottom line: It's hard to feel connected and close to someone who's tipsy or drunk. It's an effective distancer, and too much distance is destructive.

I'm occasionally asked what partners can do if their spouses are drinking too much. Unfortunately, well-funded and carefully done studies comparing various approaches to speaking with alcoholics to induce behavior change have not found a superior method.[13] I do suggest bringing it up. For a percentage of folks who drink, alcoholism is a creeping thing that sneaks up on them, and it only takes being alerted that there could be a problem for them to cut back significantly.

New lines of research are focusing on exercise as a treatment for alcoholism. Exercise appears to restore natural circadian rhythms, reduces stress, and fatigues us enough to induce sleepiness at the end of the day—reducing our need for nightly alcohol to "take the edge off."[14]

## 4-9. Give up the "silent treatment" and learn to talk it out.

My father is retired military. We were taught not to speak up. . . .
Sometimes it is important not to say anything, but sometimes
it's important to let everything out.

—RICHARD KELLEY

One of the largest studies of married couples followed 373 couples, interviewing them four times over sixteen years starting when they were first married. Researchers looked at the predictors of divorce by year sixteen (46 percent of the couples had divorced by then). In the study, there was one specific type of pattern that served as a harbinger of bad things to come. This occurred when one partner was trying to express him- or herself and listen carefully to the other spouse (the researchers called this constructive) while the other partner avoided conversation or withdrew (called withdrawal).[15] If this sounds familiar to you, tune in now.

Here's the interesting piece. The angry partners who were labeled as withdrawing actually felt that they were protecting their spouse from their anger. They were following Grandma's old adage, "If you can't say anything nice, don't say anything at all." But when researchers asked the spouses of withdrawing partners how they felt, they shared that they interpreted the silent treatment as a lack of interest.[16] The thinking appeared to be, *If they can't muster enough energy to tell me what they think, they must not care that much.*

This pattern of silencing anger can be especially toxic for women, apparently. In another study, over thirty-five hundred individuals were followed for ten years. Women who "self-silenced" during conflicts with their spouses were four times likelier to die during the study period.[17]

Speaking about what's in our hearts can be very helpful. Ever notice that people who live alone their entire lives sound strange? When we live in our own heads, we can drift away from reality. Many of us have had this experience. We're nursing along some angry or strange idea in our heads and then when we bring it up with our spouse, they dramatically change our perspective with a few words.

Richard Kelley, one of the men I interviewed, shared that for him, it took learning that his wife needed him to speak sometimes, especially when he was upset, because she could tell that something was wrong, but she had no sense of what it was. The silent treatment is lethal because it leads to self-incriminating speculations.

Some of the folks I interviewed shared that they don't like fighting when their spouse is ill, that it feels unfair to "hit them when they're down." So rather than saying anything, they are silent. Unfortunately, their spouse often knows something is wrong because of the silence. Some, like Richard, who grew up in a military family in which emotions were not discussed, had to learn how to talk to his wife about his pain, confusion, and, when appropriate, his anger. Individuals who grew up in families in which emotion was always present may feel confused with spouses who grew up in quiet households that never shared emotional upset.

I've also noticed a gender-related problem around emotions. I'm often skeptical about making wide generalizations about men and women, because my experience is that many generalizations don't hold, but I have noticed a difference in how men and women label emotions, and this is backed up by research into a phenomenon known as alexithymia. Literally translated, it means "lack of words for emotion." It does appear that men are more likely to be alexithymic than women.[18]

Many women appear to have been born with all sixty-four emotional crayons. They can label everything they feel and use words like "angst" or "sanguine" or "ornery." In contrast, many men only have the six-pack of emotional crayons. "Fine," "angry," "sad," "happy," "worried." Oh, and "confused." This inability to label every subtle emotion can impede men from talking about what they are feeling. They know they don't feel happy, but they don't have the specific words to precisely say what they mean, and they don't want to get it wrong. So they stay quiet. Meanwhile, their spouse may be thinking, *Doesn't he feel something about all this?* Or worse, *Doesn't he care?!*

In these situations, I often encourage the silent spouses to experiment with sharing what's in their heart, as accurately as they are able, but understanding that they don't have to communicate perfectly to be effective. The non-quiet spouse just needs some indication that you care and, when you're upset, to understand the cause. This is especially true when the cause is amenable to change. While silence may be easier, our research suggests that it isn't better. When normally silent spouses do share what they feel, it often opens their relationships in important ways, leading to greater intimacy, warmth, and mutual understanding.

# 5

# Having a Great Relationship during Treatment

Cancer has always felt to me like another full-time job. It requires energy and can invade other aspects of our life. So this chapter is about logistics, the details of life, and how to navigate them to protect your relationship and help you flourish together.

First, I'll share the wisdom of compartmentalizing business and romance. Then we'll examine some complex decisions for spouses, namely how to balance work with being at major medical events. We'll go over some advice about simplifying our lives, the value of exercising together, and how to navigate role changes.

The next lesson concerns food. Many couples quarrel over what the patient eats, and I have some direct advice about this. We'll also cover "chemobrain" and how couples can work together to avoid missing important information or embarrassing ourselves. Finally, I have some direct words for patients who sometimes get so absorbed in our illness worlds that we forget that cancer is happening to our spouse, too.

## 5-1. Have a weekly business meeting and a HOT ("no cancer") date night.

There was, and still is, a huge part of me that still screams to be seen as the funny, quirky, loving woman that I am.

—JANICE HALLFORD

These two recommendations go together. First, I recommend that all of the couples I work with have a business meeting once weekly. This is the time to talk about how we're going to get the radiator fixed given that this is a chemotherapy week, and decide if we will still have my brother and his family over like we'd planned before the diagnosis. How tough would it be on us if we started paying someone to mow the lawn instead of taking the time to do it ourselves, given all of the other stresses? And who's going to call the nurse to say the prescriptions are running out?

The business meetings serve many purposes. They allow us to clear our heads of life details and make plans to address potential problems. We can assign jobs to the person most able to do them best. These also proactively address stressful, argument-provoking topics when we are calm, and they help us navigate changes in roles necessitated by treatment.

Set aside a half hour, preferably at the same time every week, for the business meeting.

Here's the best part. Having a business meeting frees us up to have a no-cancer date night (or date day). By "no cancer" I mean that cancer and related information are not discussed during the date. It is, in fact, the only time I think couples should truly avoid the topic completely and just focus on fun and romance. No-cancer date nights are purely romantic events when we are engaged in something we both enjoy.

Even without cancer, it's easy for couples to get consumed by the industry of modern living. Just keeping a household functioning is a job, and given our obligations to work and family and community, many couples stop experiencing one another as romantic partners and only see one another as business partners—and now, cancer comrades. Add to this the physical changes induced by treatment—from lost hair, weight changes, and general malaise—and it's easy to see how romance is challenged.

It's also easy to become a professional cancer couple. That is, to be so focused on cancer and the battle that we lose our true identities. Date nights remind us of who we are as a couple.

Some are skeptical that this is possible. My experience has been that even in the darkest hours couples can still enjoy one another's company and a pinch of romance. Ideally, a date gets us out of the house. There's always the romantic dinner and a movie, but anything you both enjoy qualifies. Couples I've worked with or know have done no-cancer birding, antiquing, hiking, or even just going for a drive in the woods, mountains, or near water. These are times for flirting and love and these can be achieved even when energy is waning and cancer feels all around. For couples who are housebound, watching your favorite television programs together works, too.

Date nights reset our compasses. They remind us of what attracted us to our partners, they help us experience one another as lovers instead of cosurvivors, and they can reinsert laughter and fun into our lives. Experienced survivors know that just because cancer visits our lives, it doesn't mean that all of the fun and enjoyment need evaporate. It is still possible to share terrific music, feel the air after a cleansing rain, hear the sound of wind through the leaves—and see our partner laugh at our jokes, and nuzzle, and flirt.

## 5-2. Especially for lovers: Unless you are the last soldier defending the earth from alien annihilation, chances are, you can be there for major medical events. *Work less.*

She wants me to work less, but I have to keep things going. I finally compromised, and moved my law practice closer to home and worked at home some. We make less, but it was better. Still these are hard decisions.

—Terry Carliglio

He said he wanted to come to my doctor appointments, but he kept showing up late.

—Rhonda T.

Let me put this as simply as I can. I've worked in a hospital for more than twenty years and, as a result, have spent some time with dying patients and their families. Toward the end of life, we take stock of the important things and tend to search for a sense of meaning. Not once has a dying patient or lover or family member said to me, "I only wish I'd worked more."

I understand the desire to work in the midst of the cancer experience. First, we usually need the money. Second, we may fear losing our jobs in a challenging economy. Work can also be helpful psychologically. It's often one of the few places where we can feel a sense of accomplishment and that we are doing something observable to help. That feeling of being helpful is often evasive during cancer.

I don't want to oversimplify this. Some of these decisions are hard: Should I go with my husband to meet his radiation oncologist or meet with the buyers who may help us finally close a deal? Should I stay home with her when she's feeling ill or pull another shift? Should I quit this job even if I have seniority here, if I can get one closer to home and start over as the new girl?

One way to think about decisions regarding which visits to attend is to estimate the importance of each medical visit. Not all medical visits are the same. Some are big. These are the ones where we're making major decisions, getting big news, or dealing with frightening symptoms or side effects. It's almost always important to be together during these times. There are also small visits, when we're picking up a prescription, having a single radiation treatment, or checking on the healing of a surgical wound. That said, we sometimes disagree about the importance or intensity of a meeting. As the patient, there were times when I felt intense vulnerability and wanted someone with me, even though the seriousness of the visit was not great. Just stepping into a hospital or clinic can *feel* big.

Over the five years that I was ill, someone went with me to every one of my chemotherapy treatments, every surgery, and every procedure. Usually it was Terry. Sometimes it was my parents, and a few times friends helped out. I went to the radiation treatments alone. We did the same with Terry. I was there for every one of her chemo treatments but not for all of her radiation treatments or her meetings with her plastic surgeon.

In general, and this is for the lovers, err toward being there with the patient in your life. When we're sick we feel more vulnerable, and this is the nectar of the human experience. To feel that when the assault is on the way, there's someone with us in the foxhole. To hold our heads. To rub our necks. To stand with us against the winds.

## 5-3. Wherever possible, simplify and reduce the stress at home.

Our kids were young. The three that lived at home were fourteen, twelve, and eleven. Bill took them aside one time, after they knew what was going on, and told them that they really needed to pull together and take stress off of Mommy. He told them two of the things that stressed me most were arguing and yelling at each other and not cleaning their rooms. The kids went out of their way to clean their rooms and take their arguments, which are inevitable in kids that age, outside.

—Becky M. Olson

Here's a short list of things couples told me they did to simplify and reduce stress during illness. First, many tried to stop arguing and even minor bickering. The topics are usually not important, but included arguing about television, the thermostat, directions, spending, and vacations with the spouse's children, in-laws, or loud friends.

They reduced work hours or adjusted their jobs; some reduced volunteer activities (others increased them). They ate out more often, carried food in, or bought—*gasp!*—frozen or other easy-to-make meals. They were more selective about housework: keeping things clean to avoid infections but not necessarily as tidy. So they kept up with changing air-conditioner filters, keeping soap in the dispensers, and vacuuming but allowed some regular maintenance items to slip: mowing lawns once every ten days instead of once or twice weekly, wearing some clothing twice instead of once, and waiting to get the trash out until the bins were completely full.

The trick is to balance activities that will bring a sense of purpose, welcomed distraction, and enjoyment against those that are depleting and cause more stress than they are worth. I want you to be connected to other people and to things that are good for your head and mercilessly slice away the rest.

Some readers are inevitably the type who have never said "no" their entire lives. That is, whenever someone in the community or family has a need, they come to you for help, volunteering, counsel, or protection. Here is an ideal opportunity to learn this new skill. Saying "no" occasionally can help you protect valuable energy. It can ensure that you are with your spouse instead of helping someone else when you are needed.

Simplifying also requires conversation. Some activities are more fun for one of you than the other, or may be more important. Talk and make decisions as a couple.


## 5-4. Exercise together.

He pushes me—we have gone up to the clubhouse to walk on the treadmill even though I can only walk for five minutes, and last night we walked down the street even though it was very hot.

But he says, "You need to walk, you need to get up, if you are not going to walk outside you are going to walk the length of the house ten times." And I better do it because he will come back and say, "Have you done this yet?"

—JoAnn McClure

For years, oncologists told newly diagnosed patients with cancer to rest and "take it easy," and indeed, some studies show that as many as half of all oncologists are still recommending rest. But the data on exercise in survivorship is overwhelmingly against this advice. In fact, there are now a number of cancer survivors who are also doctoral-level researchers who are showing that this advice is dead wrong.

Anna Schwartz is among them. Dr. Schwartz was diagnosed with lymphoma when she was a nursing student in 1988. She initially suffered from depression and said she felt completely overwhelmed by the diagnosis. She decided to try exercise and began cycling with a local group of riders. At first, she was disappointed that she couldn't keep up with them and worked hard to improve her cycling so she could perform as they did. She didn't realize at first that these riders were among cycling's elite, including Olympic gold medalists and national champions. Eventually, she could keep up with them, and ultimately she landed three world records is less than five years, including cycling 418 miles in twenty-four hours. Straight. She did this during her on-again, off-again treatment for what she called "my little problem." Her cancer.

Dr. Schwartz went on to get a doctoral degree in nursing and focus all of her research on the role of exercise in cancer survivorship. Her work and the work of many others have shown that while fatigue and pain are common complaints during and after the cancer experience, exercise can have a profound impact.

Exercise doesn't just improve what researchers call "quality of life." It also appears that exercise should be considered a treatment. For example, for breast cancer patients, recent research shows that exercising two and a half hours per week reduces a woman's chances of dying or suffering a recurrence by 40 percent.[1] That's a more impressive improvement than many other treatments. The risk reduction in men with prostate cancer was also an impressive 46 percent.[2] (Breast and prostate cancer are the most commonly studied diseases because they are the most frequently diagnosed illnesses, and researchers typically need large number of patients to draw conclusions. I'm sure exercise is just as helpful for patients with other cancers.)

Even just four weeks of gentle exercise, such as hatha yoga, significantly enhances quality of life in patients by improving sleep and reducing fatigue.[3] Walking programs such as those that have been long recommended by the journalist, cancer survivor, and race walker Carolyn Scott Kortge (and studied by a number of researchers including Karen Basen-Engquist and her colleagues at the M.D. Anderson Cancer Center) also improve pain and improve overall ratings of health.

There are some precautions worth considering. At the height of treatment, there is nothing wrong with taking a little time off to recover. And patients with severe, acute anemia should wait to exercise to avoid undue strain on their hearts (those with chronic anemia can habituate to exercise). Folks with osteoporosis should discuss exercise with their doctor and start weight-bearing exercise. Those with nerve damage, depending on the damage, might be unable to do some exercises without pain.

Let's talk about couples and exercise. Couples I interviewed fell into two categories, the active and the nonactive. The active couples typically had at least one member who was an "activity engine," who demanded, required, and insisted that the couple do activities that required some physical action, from walking to more vigorous cycling, aerobic classes, swimming, or even sports. Sometimes these activities were as simple and low-key as walking in the local mall during inclement weather or doing activities at home using video programs available through YouTube on the Internet, on-demand cable television programs, or DVDs.

One woman I spoke with, JoAnn McClure, shared that after breast cancer, and then colon and rectal cancer that resulted in her getting a colostomy bag, she felt fatigued. "Usually I just lie on the couch because it feels good," she told me. In her case, it was her husband who hounded her to get up and move, and he often would exercise with her. He demanded that they leave the house every day. When I interviewed her, she told me, "Today was 'all the way to the Dollar General Store.' You have to just do something."

The nonactive couples had never been particularly active or the active member of the couple was now the one who felt lazy and fatigued. In those cases, it was very difficult to get motivated. Yet this is the precise time when it makes sense to do so.

The beginning of any exercise regimen is the hardest, and here are critical points. First, start slowly enough! Walking or chair exercises are a good place to start. For some, exercising in a pool makes sense, as the buoyancy makes it easier to move.

Second, do it together. For a while (well after treatment), Terry and I did calisthenics while watching movies on television. We eventually escalated and did an entire, popular, and rigorous exercise program known as P90X, which helped us both lose weight and tone up as we exercised for between fifty minutes and an hour every day for three months. Looking back, we were mostly encouraging of each other, though she occasionally pointed out my poor form or made fun of how unlimber I am. If we can survive these mild indignities, we can enjoy the many benefits of exercise.

Finally, stick to it. A bit every day.

## 5-5. Bring extreme patience to role changes.

I am teaching him how to cook and clean and how to not put bleach in the clothing (we had a few splotches). I think he is going to be a good cook and he cleans the house. He didn't realize what I did all these years.

—JoAnn McClure

When I came home from having my lymph node surgery, it was lunchtime and I was standing there making my husband's lunch. My daughter walked in the door and said, "Dad, you see anything wrong with this picture?" and he said, "No!" (Laughs)

—Barbara Janzen

When I was ten I was the ring bearer at my aunt's wedding. Later, relieved to not have dropped or lost the ring, I was sitting with my brother at one of the huge circular tables while everyone danced. My uncle Samuel wandered over, and I remember the disco ball throwing little circles of light across his forehead after he dropped down next to us.

After a few pleasantries he looked at my brother and me and said, "Here's the most important advice I have about girlfriends. Are you listening?" I nodded and then elbowed my seven-year-old brother, who looked up at him.

"Never, ever, ever. Not ever. Are you listening? Don't ever yourself try to teach your girl how to drive a manual transmission. Especially not in your 1968 GT 350 Mustang convertible." Then he took a deep breath as if he had just ascended after an incredibly deep pearl dive and quivered a little.

Cancer often necessitates couples having to change household jobs. During the interview process for this book, I asked a number of couples if they'd had role changes induced by cancer. In a number of cases, this question was met with an awkward silence and then a story that involved yelling, clicked tongues, or eye rolling.

For example, couples I interviewed taught one another how to pay bills online, vacuum, mow the lawn, and my favorite: back up a boat trailer. Not all of these transitions had gone perfectly. It is startling to realize how much patience we can show our friends— or even our pets!—when teaching them something new, but how little reserve we sometimes have for our lovers.

When tasked with teaching one's spouse how to do something that is new for them, I often ask the teacher in the relationship to imagine that they are back during the romantic early part of their relationship. This sometimes helps members of the couple muster the patience they need.

That said, here are a few rules for the teacher.

1. No taking over. When my wife uses the remote control on the television she is slow. Seasons pass while she clicks to where she needs to be. She prefers to gradually peruse the menu options, carefully reading each option before making a decision. I, in contrast, know where the channels are that I'm planning to reach and directly punch in the numbers. In truth, it takes my wife about three seconds longer to get to where we need to be than when I'm in command, and while it's true that I'm never going to get those seconds of my life back, the consequences if I grab the remote and announce, "Just let me do it!" (sound familiar, anyone?) are far worse than if I sit quietly. The same is true if we are talking about how to do the laundry, pay the bills, or back up a boat. If our spouse hasn't done something dangerous, let them muddle through; all of us are imperfect when we're learning a new skill.

2. You are allowed two encouraging phrases for every bit of technical advice about a task. Ever watch a talented gymnastics or Little League coach work with the kids who aren't naturals? They are incredibly encouraging. For each word of technical advice they give, like "Watch the ball" or "Keep your back straight," they give two encouraging phrases like "That's it!" or "Nice job" or "You're getting it" or "That was better."

3. Accept that for most tasks, there's more than one way to get it done. A friend of mine, Dr. Lisa Sinz, runs a medical simulation laboratory. The lab focuses on teaching health trainees how to

do various medical tasks, from flushing a PICC line (simple) to intubating a patient (complex). She's noticed that even for the simple tasks, many health professionals have the way they do it, and they all believe the way they do it is absolutely right and *often the only way*. "But you know what?" she shared with me. "They all work." Chances are good that your spouse will do tasks differently from you. That's OK. That can still work.

On the other side of the equation, the learner often has to tolerate not knowing how to do something well immediately. It's amazing how many adults have successfully avoided learning to do something new for years! As a result, we sometimes have little patience for ourselves when we don't do a task perfectly the first time. Some tasks have changed over time on us, too. Consider the average modern washing machine. Unlike bygone eras when washers had one dial and a starting button, the modern washer may have a hundred possible combinations and may appear, at first, more like flying a jet than cleaning a pair of jeans.

Unlike past eras when we all balanced checkbooks, now many of us bank online and instead of adding columns, the task requires understanding how to navigate software menus. Basic life tasks can be difficult, and it's important to be patient with ourselves (and our spouses).

## 5-6. Don't fight over food.

I was cooking for Nancy. That may have been worse for our health than the cancer.

—Bob N.

It was the first time I saw him panic. You know, he's usually . . . very, very calm, but when I hit the wall and just wouldn't eat anything, he got really distressed.

—NANCY N.

Food is a powerful part of many of our lives. Many of us start our relationships in the company of food. We take one another to dinner. We cook for each other. We talk about our favorite foods and desserts. In the Broadway play *A House of Blue Leaves*, the female lead is willing to have sex before marriage, but she won't cook for her husband until they are married. Instead, she shows him a photo album of the many splendid dishes she can cook. He's hooked.

At restaurants you can tell when a couple is intensifying their flirtation if they share food, and especially if they physically feed one another. A fork offered across the table is a sure sign that the ember of romance is burning brightly.

When I was a first-year graduate student I was accustomed to cooking ramen noodles and microwavable frozen packages. Pot pies, lasagna, and other horrible plastic foods. I'd dated a few other graduate students whose culinary expertise was similar to mine. But then I met Terry, who offered to make me dinner. We sat in her little house eating around a real table with a real tablecloth and real dishes. She served a chicken cacciatore with glazed string beans and Cuban rice. Steam lingered from the serving dishes and she wore an apron with "Queen of the Kitchen" emblazoned across it in bright block letters. It was spectacular.

Food is also a powerful part of our heritage. Our cultures offer "our" foods—the foods we grew up eating, that our grandparents may have eaten. They tie us to our families and our backgrounds, our history. Many families routinely have family dinners where our most important family conversations occur.

Food is also about comfort. During times of crisis or after a death, communities often bring food. When Terry was diagnosed with cancer, a colleague of mine from work arranged for a pleasant stream of home-cooked meals to come to the house.

Perhaps it should be no surprise then that when our eating habits change during treatment—increasing or decreasing—it can deeply impact our spouses. Food is one of the few areas of our lives where we feel we have control, and some have argued that we can fight cancer with food or harm ourselves with the wrong foods.

In fact, there is data to support the notion that dietary changes can impact cancers that already exist. For example, Gerald Krystal, a research scientist in British Columbia, studied mice implanted with cancer cells (I know, harsh, right?) and then fed them one of two diets. The first diet was roughly one-half carbohydrates, one-quarter protein, and one-quarter fat. Then he and his colleagues fed a second group a diet of more than one-half protein, one-quarter fat, and less than one-quarter carbs. The second group of mice did far better.

In fact, 70 percent of the mice on the first diet died of cancer, while only 30 percent in the second group died of cancer (and more than half of the mice on the second diet who had cancer lived a normal lifespan).[4] Krystal and his colleagues present a very simple hypothesis: that cancer cells need fuel in the form of glucose (sugar), and the high-protein diet starves cancer cells of needed sugars. Others have argued that the type of protein is important, with plant-based proteins being more helpful than meat-based proteins, which may increase the risk of lung or colorectal cancers.

Some couples mentioned fish oil to me, so I include a brief paragraph here. Fish oil's advantage is that it includes omega-3 fatty acids (as do walnuts),[5] especially a substance known as DHA (docosahexaenoic acid), for which there is early evidence of reduced leukocytosis, systematic inflammation, and oxidative stress, which are all processes involved in the growth of tumors.[6] While there have been some exciting findings, large meta-analyses have found mixed results for omega-3s in general, and their impact on cancer incidence and growth, or mortality, remains questionable.[7]

The following foods have all been recommended for cancer prevention or treatment: beans, berries, green vegetables, flaxseed, garlic, grapes, tea (especially green tea), soy (though soy is a phytoestrogen, its impact on estrogenergic breast cancer is not understood), tomatoes, and whole grains. Despite those recommendations, the data have lagged behind; aside from the studies listed above, and information about the known dangers of obesity, there aren't clear scientific findings yet about connections between specific food choices and cancer. We suspect highly processed meats may worsen cancer, but we don't yet have solid evidence.

Unfortunately, making dietary changes when cancer and cancer treatments have already assaulted how our food tastes, changed our appetite, and limited our ability to have fun in other ways creates a recipe (ha ha) for problems. After surgeries, the drugs used to combat pain (like morphine) can slow our bowels, causing bloating and reducing our appetite. Mouth sores from immune-system assaulting chemotherapy can make eating painful. Radiation can change our saliva secretions, drying our mouths, and may also cause nausea, vomiting, or diarrhea.

Patients with gastrointestinal malignancies face additional dietary challenges. Tumors in the stomach or intestines can alter how the body uses some nutrients, causing a challenging situation in that the patient will appear to eat enough food, but the body will not absorb the nutrients from the food.

Some drugs make swallowing difficult. Radiation to the neck or mouth (or total body irradiation) can increase mouth secretions by inflaming salivary glands. And those of us who have had chemotherapy or some forms of head and neck radiation know that treatment can impact our taste buds. As my interviewee JoAnn McClure said, "Everything tastes like sawdust!"

Finally, patients with advanced cancers will almost always lose their desire to eat. Patients with lung cancers, pancreatic cancers, or gastrointestinal cancers may also develop a cluster of symptoms known as cachexia, which describes the loss of appetite plus weight loss, muscle loss, and severe fatigue. Consulting with a nutritionist who understands cancer and who can offer dietary supplementation can be helpful.

Unfortunately, fighting over food is common among couples. For our entire lives, our relationship with food has been something we've controlled. So it's natural for spouses to believe that patients can still control the way they eat and desperately want them to improve consumption. Spouses sometimes see a loss of appetite as "giving up" rather than as a predictable side effect.

*I urge you not to fight, nag, or harass one another about food.* It's destructive, it rarely results in improved appetite, and it demonstrates to the patient that the spouse has little conception of the real challenges of the disease. Having been through profound appetite loss, I can tell you that no amount of coaxing can bring it back.

For many couples, eating together is essential togetherness time, and the change in appetite can result in feelings of disconnection, as couples spend the time they used to spend together doing things apart—one spouse of a woman with ovarian cancer shared that he ate dinner while she "surfed eBay." I do urge couples to continue to spend quality time together, but occasionally it needs to be time out of the kitchen and perhaps after the spouse's dinner. This can be disorienting when our habits have been cemented in years of doing the meal preparation and cleanup together around favorite, familiar foods.

If you go on websites written by people who have never had chemotherapy or radiation themselves, they will recommend never eating spicy, sweet, or fatty foods. While I tend to agree that the cancer experience is a great time to evaluate one's diet and learn to eat great-tasting food that is also healthy, it is also true that food is more than fuel. Food can be reward, romance, distraction. When I lost my taste buds I loved spicy foods because I could taste them! In fact, I developed my fascination with hot sauces following a particularly nasty bit of chemotherapy.

Bob N.'s response to his wife's loss of appetite worked for her. She said, "I would eat five tablespoons and I would be totally full. I couldn't even think of putting another spoonful in. . . . He would say, 'OK, I'm going to put it downstairs and if you feel like eating it later I will microwave it and bring it back up.'"

An additional tension exists at the other end of the spectrum, when patients gain weight. Consider this story.

Terry walks out of the cancer center as if she has just been paroled, squinting into the Arizona sun. I have the car waiting. She climbs into the minivan, chewing a lip, and I bet she's nauseous. I can viscerally remember that feeling from after chemotherapy. Best to get her home as quickly as possible so she can lie down and relax. I put the car in gear and we pull up to the intersection that leads out of the hospital.

"Cheeseburger," she says.

Huh?

"Stop at McTrashalds."

"Really?"

"I want a huge cheeseburger. Two maybe."

"You just had chemo, aren't you nauseous?"

"Yeah. So what. I want a cheeseburger."

Like many of the women I know, Terry is extremely conscious of her weight. We try to eat relatively healthy food and particularly avoid fast food. We haven't been to a McTrashalds in years.

"Light's green." She points.

We drive up Campbell Avenue toward Fort Lowell where a large McTrashalds awaits. I expect her to change her mind. "You know, the chemo's going to kick in later, you're going to feel worse. There's a salad place just over on—"

"Don't miss the turn. Don't turn too early! You're going to miss the turn," she says. I pull into the drive-through lane. Terry leans over and surveys the menu.

When the speaker chokes awake and a disembodied voice asks for our order, Terry is quick: "Give me a double cheeseburger, large fries, large diet Coke, and chocolate shake." Then she looks at me. "You want anything?"

Two pork pops, a beef swirl, meat on a stick, and a house-sized steak.

"Uh. I guess a little hamburger."

"He'll take the double-cheeseburger," she says loudly, in case the microphone is underwater. Then she says softly, "Look, if I'm putting all of these toxins that I hate into my body, my liver won't care if I add a few more that I love, just for good measure."

This logic makes no sense. Hell, I've been working for years with an integrative medicine program that seeks to combine the best of conventional and alternative medicine. Diet is one of the primary things we seek to change. And she knows all of this; she's been a nutrition expert for years. And, truth be told, I'm a little nervous that our car might be spotted in the drive-through lane by one of my yoga-guru-diet self-actualized colleagues.

"Quit looking like I burned down your ashram and pay the girl," Terry says.

I pay the girl. In exchange, the girl hands me a large bag of toxic treats and leans over with Terry's shake, using both hands to deliver it into the Odyssey. The cup won't fit in any of our cup holders because it's large enough to have a diving board. We finally pull out and I'm relieved because at least now, as I prepare to merge into the traffic, I can pretend that we got lost if we're spotted.

Now we're out on the road, and happy eating sounds emanate from Terry's rough location. "I've worried about this stuff my whole adult life and look at me. Breast cancer. So every now and then, we're visiting the dark (muffled) . . . oh, this is good," she says, as wonderful, factory-produced smells fill the inside of the vehicle and a bag of french fries is balanced on the overturned purple sandbox bucket I brought in case she got nauseous.

I had protests. I wanted her to do everything she could to fight the cancer, and diet was part of that. But she needed to enjoy her body as it was changing, and perhaps not speaking up for once was the smartest thing I could have done.

It's true that many patients gain weight during treatment. Chemotherapy in particular frequently reduces activity levels and changes metabolism. While not ideal for health, this must be balanced against the disruptive relationship impact of fighting over weight.

## 5-7. Deal with chemobrain proactively.

At this point I was just in a fog, putting one foot in front of the other.

—LINDA SPENCE

You have the chemobrain thing, so you know, I would come out of the office and I would say, "Now did he say such and such?" So it was good he was listening.

—PRISCILLA LABONTE

Whenever he is confused I try to protect him from anyone seeing that. I don't know why exactly, but it is like I don't want them to feel bad and I don't want him to realize later there was an uncomfortable situation.

—JODY PRICE

On a windy winter day in Palo Alto, I recall walking with my wife into the chemotherapy suite at Stanford and introducing myself to the man in the chair next to mine, who squinted at me in confusion. *He's an odd one,* I thought. My wife nudged me in the ribs. "What?" I asked, "I'm just being friendly."

"You spent an hour talking to him yesterday! It's Jeff! Remember?"

I did not remember. Ativan, a drug I'd taken before getting chemotherapy, had ablated my memory for the entire day. And, obviously, embarrassed my wife.

Known as "chemobrain" by patients, the proposed mechanisms are not clearly understood. Vascular injury, inflammatory insult, toxicity to neural cells used by structures playing key roles in sensation, memory, and processing speed have all been implicated, but this is a notoriously difficult area for researchers to study. And regardless of how these mechanisms function, the reality is clear—many chemotherapy drugs and the medications we use to address the side effects of chemotherapy interfere with clear thinking.

Drugs like hydroxyurea, high-dose ifosfamide, and methotrexate are infamous for this, but there are others, too, like high-dose interleukin-2 and interferon. Medications administered to help us deal with the side effects of chemotherapy—like Ativan that day—or other drugs used to treat pain, sleep disorders, cardiac issues, or stomach problems, can also be disorienting.

There are also physical conditions common to the cancer experience that can induce confusion. Insomnia is probably the biggest culprit. Lack of sleep can be disorienting (and is a stress magnifier—insomnia can make everything worse). Other common experiences include dehydration, having too much calcium or too little sodium, anemia, heart issues, blood infections, thyroid conditions, or endocrine disorders. Obviously, when cancer gets into the brain it can also cause disorienting symptoms.

Then, of course, there's stress itself. We know that when we are stressed and worried, the amount of RAM we have available for other thinking diminishes. We lose our keys, forget phone numbers, and words may elude us.

Serious, enduring cognitive changes should be evaluated. But some confusion during the experience is normal.[8] And remember, just because you're confused doesn't mean that something horrible is happening in your brain. It's more likely chemobrain—a temporary set of cognitive changes. Just because chemobrain is common, of course, doesn't mean it won't drive our spouses crazy.

I strongly advise coping as a couple. First, write things down. Keep one notebook and track medications, side effects, and insurance information. Pillboxes can also be very helpful when we are confused. In serious situations, we may need help with cooking and driving. Clearly, meeting with physicians and nurses together can be helpful. A soft-spoken man from Maryland named Ted Kennedy shared that his wife, a patient, was often quiet in meetings with physicians because the entire experience seemed overwhelming. He suggested, "Go with a pad of paper every time you meet with doctors and nurses, don't be afraid to ask questions."

As much as possible, stick to a routine. Keep your keys, wallet/purse/man-purse, and shoes in the same place. When we are confused, having routine can assist us. Our routine should include getting enough physical activity and sleep.

Slow down. Quit the multitasking. No more talking on the

phone while driving, no matter how "hands free" your automobile. Don't eat while doing the bills. Focusing on one task at a time can help us stay on top of things when we are prone to confusion.

Leave one another alone. In the midst of the stress of the cancer experience, we can feel frustrated when our spouses forget things. This can be especially trying when we are in the midst of juggling treatment and the rest of life's challenges—which don't stop just because cancer has visited. Bills that don't get paid, forgotten voice messages, and lost keys are the most common complaints I heard during interviews. These are hard for spouses because they ended up causing more work in rescheduled appointments, time spent searching for lost objects, or frantic calls to utilities to avoid shutoff. But obviously, these were not done on purpose. Expressing frustration just amplifies the problem.

Finally—and this one is hard—ask for help when you need it. If there are friends or loved ones available to help with concrete tasks (bill paying, for example) during a phase when confusion reigns, this is a time to ask them. This is often difficult for us, because we are usually trading our privacy and control for assistance, but if "my squash ain't working" as one patient put it, "borrow someone else's."

It's OK to have a sense of humor about these things. One woman sitting next to us in the waiting room told us that that her spouse, a patient, was lucky. She nudged her head in his direction and he shook his head, as if to say, *Not this story again.*

"The chemotherapy confused him so much that he lit our house on fire when he forgot that he was cooking."

I asked, "How was that lucky?!"

He looked over at us, "The water from the bath I'd forgotten I was running upstairs came down through the ceiling and put it out, no problem." His hand hovered in the air, batting down gently, as if snuffing a fire. Then they laughed together.

## 5-8. For patients: It isn't only about you.

Cancer is not something that happens to one person, it happens to couples.

—Penny Carruth

Sometimes people get so, so caught up with "this is all about me, everyone has to be with me" and they forget there are other things that need to go on.

—Helen Kelley

Sometimes you feel a little guilt because you are the well one.

—Jody Price

It's been tough. I don't like to leave him. I don't like to leave his side. I have taken a few breaks. It's OK.

—Valree Milson

Let me say this as clearly as I can to all the patients out there. Just because you're the one suffering through the physical challenges doesn't mean you are the only one suffering. Having played both roles, neither is fun. Cancer is happening to the support too, and they need to be able to get their water bottles along the way if they are going to hold up throughout the marathon. This is not a trivial issue.

The cancer experience is typically fluid, meaning that we don't spend all of our time in the same exact physical or psychological state over time. The day we received chemotherapy or the day after might be miserable and flu-like, but three days later we might feel absolutely fine. Depressive swings can drive us to our knees one day, and then the next we might feel hopeful and energized.

Some of this is predictable as we get further into the experience, and some doesn't follow a pattern. When we feel horrible, we may want and feel that we need our spouse to be with us physically and emotionally. But when we feel well, we may be fully prepared to be at work or be completely independent.

Some patients respond to these vicissitudes by demanding that their spouse be with them, or attentive, at all times. This can be crippling. And let's face it, life goes on. Someone has to go grocery shopping. Driver's licenses expire and need renewal, the fan in the bathroom may need repair. And there's work and finances.

Ideally, we patients have our spouse's attention through the hardest parts, and during the periods when we feel better, we give them the independence they need to help us keep the household going, get to work, and to enjoy some of their time doing favorite activities.

Caregivers I spoke with who were getting too few breaks were miserable. They sounded like they needed caregivers themselves. Some had physical symptoms including headaches, back pain, neck pain, digestion issues, and even visual field changes. Others had insomnia, concentration problems, low energy, and changes in appetite.

And in every case, the patient had *no idea* their spouse had these symptoms. Here's a representative quote from an anonymous husband of a patient being treated for ovarian cancer:

"Are you kidding, given everything she's suffered through? A little pain won't kill me. I can't tell her about this crap, she's got enough going on." And yet, when caregivers run themselves down, they are no good to anyone. This is not abstract; a number of caregivers shared that they had, for a time, become nonfunctional from exhaustion. In the words of Nana, my grandmother: "If you are tired you should sleep more. If you are hungry you should eat more."

As I've just mentioned, cancer is a marathon and both members need to get their water bottles along the way. But that's often easier said than done. "There are things to do! People we love to protect and take care of!" And maybe guilt gets in the way too: "It's not fair for me to feel this fine when the love of my life is suffering!"

There are a number of other factors that interfere with caregivers getting the help they need. The first are perspective and scale. It's difficult to focus on getting one's teeth cleaned when your spouse is going through chemotherapy. We think: *How can I bother with these trivialities when there are such huge things happening in our lives?* And yet, physical maintenance is still important.

The reality is, both jobs are incredibly hard, and each job has pain. But we cannot allow that pain to prevent us from getting our jobs done. And one of our jobs as caregivers is taking care of ourselves well enough that we can function. The job requires focus, organization, and memory: without self-care, all of these skills suffer.

Caregivers may need to explain to their spouse with cancer that they need a break. Some breaks are micro, as in, "I'm frying a little here, I just need a walk and I'll be back in an hour refreshed and good to go." Others may be more major and take a few days away, as in, "I've asked your sister to come in for a few days. I'm going to visit with my brother and get some exercise and clear my head, so I can come back to you good as new."

A little attention from the ill spouse can go a long way. In the midst of her treatment, my wife occasionally asked me how *I* was doing. It was a little jarring, and tender, and buoyed me in a way that nothing else could. Her understanding that the experience was happening to both of us made it easier. When I was ill, I was less mature and more self-centered than she was. I don't remember ever asking how she was. Nor my parents, who struggled mightily, I understood later.

6

# Work Together to Get What You Need from Outside People

When we are facing a crisis, the people in our lives can be supportive or destructive, and sometimes both. Learning to navigate our social environment can teach us how to invite help from the right people and manage those who lack the skills to be helpful. There are also those people in our lives who are just difficult. When we're ill we may lack the ability to cope with people who suck our life force away. Sometimes fighting cancer requires that we clear out noxious relationships that drain us of important energy. This can be painful, and I'll share some examples.

While engaging with our social groups can be wonderfully rewarding, it also invites the question of how much information to share. While researching this book, I met many couples who disagreed—and in a few cases, spouses felt that they had been betrayed when private information was discussed. There are benefits and costs associated with other people understanding the intimate details of some of our treatments, and I'll try to provide some criteria to help you work together in advance to decide what to tell whom.

We turn next to support groups, both in person and online. I'll get into the ambivalence that some people, especially men, feel about support groups and try to unpack which parts of this make sense, and what's lost if you completely shut out other people who have been through the same challenges you face.

The last part of the chapter addresses the difficulty many people have accepting needed help, even though learning to do so can be a critical skill.

## 6-1. Not all well-meaning people in your lives have the ability or skills to be supportive in the ways you need.

People amaze you. People amazed me. I didn't always get it where I expected it either. And sometimes where I expected it I didn't get it at all.

—LINDA SPENCE

We were back and forth to Baltimore a lot. I worked at a high school before I retired, in maintenance. I was out of that school two years, and one Sunday the secretary came to this house with an envelope. Those teachers gave me over $500 for gas.

—HARMAN SPENCE

I had a young lady who worked with me and I'm telling you she was a godsend. About three days after I would take the chemo I would come in and I would be stiff and I would be almost in tears and she'd put on music and she would get a book of poetry. I'm telling you, she would have the kids draw pictures, just anything that would take me from that ugly place where I was into someplace that was bright and sunshiny.

—SANDRA WHITAKER

Just because someone in your life has decent intentions doesn't mean they have skills. While we were sick, we heard a variety of comments from well-intentioned people that were challenging to hear. "My uncle Bob had Hodgkin's disease just like you. Uh. He died." Or, "You're lucky."

Other people can influence you as a couple. Friends and acquaintances and work connections can all play a role in how well you navigate the experience. And, there's a big difference between sympathy and real connection. Let me demonstrate:

Terry and I are shopping at the Too-Expensive-for-Words supermarket. She's had her surgical reconstruction, but chemotherapy is still one week away. The supermarket has mostly the same things as the Safeway supermarket near our house, but here the produce is displayed on doilies and there are mahogany shelves and long rows of clean glass cases with special lights. We would both rather be at Trader Joe's across town, but the pesto is good and Terry has a few other unique ingredients she's looking for.

"If I'm only cooking once a week, I want it to be special," she has proclaimed.

While grazing through the organic cereal aisle, where one can find breakfast food that can also be used as packing material or wall insulation, I hear Terry squeal a greeting. Glancing over, I see Terry and a woman I don't recognize squeaking at one another in an octave best left to dogs and bats. They obviously know each other well, from work I imagine.

I continue looking for a cereal that will taste good, has something modestly healthy, but won't cost me a five-spot. Then, out of the corner of my eye I see Terry clutch the woman's hand and start to walk in the opposite direction.

"Hey," I yell out.

"Oh," she says, "I'm just going to show Ellen my results." It takes me a moment to translate. She's just said, *I'm going to show this woman my new breasts.* I haven't seen the new breasts myself. But now my wife is wandering toward the back of the supermarket, through the double swinging doors and into some high-end supermarket bathroom to reveal her boobs to a coworker.

I imagine myself after a prostate surgery running into Francisco in the supermarket.

"Hey, come on, Francisco, let me show you the fine job the surgeon did right between the twins and my back door."

I wander aimlessly through the cheese section, where four thousand cheeses in various sizes are available for adoption. And the coffee aisle, where a second mortgage will get you coffee beans that were individually nurtured to maturity in South America by owner-operators.

Terry and her friend reappear near the wines.

"Great result," her friend says to me. "You must be very pleased."

"Oh, I am. I'm quite proud," I say, as if we're discussing Alexandra winning the Nobel prize for second graders. The woman smiles, pats me on the shoulder, and disappears into the spice aisle.

"Her result wasn't quite as good," Terry says to me. On seeing my face, she adds, "Yeah, she had breast cancer, too. She saw Mc-Naulty."

"So you two stood in the bathroom and showed each other? Why wasn't I invited? When I was in tenth grade I dreamed of being around for that sort of thing," I say. Terry has learned to ignore these sorts of observations.

"This is a good place to get mangoes. Go get us some mangoes." She prods. And I am sent away.

In truth, I don't know of another area of oncology where patients routinely share in this way. But as Terry walks through the supermarket, she seems buoyed. Now we find each other back in the frozen-food section, or at least that's what I think it is when you have food in cardboard boxes kept at freezing temperatures, though the sign reads, "Premade Gourmet Meals." This reminds me of when we call used cars "preowned." Another woman I don't know approaches us and I'm anticipating more playful banter.

"Terry?" The woman's face goes white. Her neck cranes forward slowly. "How . . . how ARE you?" Her face is scrunched in concentration as if she is about to memorize a twenty-digit bank safe code.

"Uh," Terry says, "OK." At least I was until you did that thing with your neck, her face reveals.

"OK? Really? Oh, well good. Oh, you two have been through so much. Oh, this must be Dan," she says. She says this looking at me, the portrait of angst and sympathy. I wonder if we just survived a flood no one told me about.

"How are the kids?"

"Fine," Terry says.

To avoid the woman, I feign looking for a meal. "Confetti Rice Pilaf & Chicken with Honey BBQ Sauce" has a bright box. Next to it, a company by Moosewood puts out a Moroccan stew that also looks appetizing. Or perhaps "Farfalle Spinach with Pesto Sauce."

"So, of course, you're buying frozen food. Makes sense," the woman says, nodding.

"No, actually, I was going to make dinner," Terry says.

"Right," I say. Both of them are looking at me.

"Well," the woman says, "I'm so sorry for both of you." And she smirks a sad smirk and walks on down the aisle.

As we shuffle away from the woman, I can tell Terry is sinking beneath the grim weight of her sympathy. I want to re-create the playfulness she had moments ago when she showed a relative stranger her breasts, but the moment is gone. I almost offer to let her show me her new breasts in the supermarket bathroom, but with rare restraint, I manage to keep my mouth shut, just this once.

People want to be supportive, and we don't have great social rules for what to say. I'm convinced that this woman in the store wanted to be helpful and caring, but instead, she came off as an incredible downer because she led with her sympathy. When people don't know what to do I'd suggest asking where in the process the patient is, and then talking about normal stuff. As in, "Hey, I heard you were doing chemo soon, how's that going?" And then, "Did you hear that Ann Jones lit herself on fire with a curling iron? She's fine, but the curling iron didn't make it." Don't ask,

"How are you?" Because it leads to what a breast cancer veteran and a friend of mine, Kathy LaTour, once called "Fine Syndrome." There are fifty different ways to say "I'm fine" when we aren't.

Terry needed to be around people who could make her laugh and treat her as if she were still normal, even if she didn't always feel normal. And I had to learn how to steer her toward friends who would make her feel good, and away from ones who might do that, you know, that weird sympathy thing with their necks.

Try to surround yourselves with people who can provide what you need psychologically. Sometimes that means that your social network will shift. The friends you've had that matched you well before cancer are not always the same ones who will match you well now. For this reason, we turn to the next lesson, which focuses on clearing out destructive relationships.

## 6-2. Sometimes we need to clear out other relationships that have been causing stress in our marriages.

You need to take stock. Sometimes that means clearing away relationships from people who don't have your back. I had to limit my mother. She's very unhappy and it always caused stress in my marriage. I just had to let her be unhappy.

—CLARE KENNEDY

Life doesn't stop when cancer visits. When we enter the rapids of the cancer experience, some of the folks aboard our life's ship may not be the people we would have chosen to help us navigate a life crisis. But worse, in some cases, those people fail to see the crisis in our lives and continue to drain us of valuable resources, energy, and focus.

In the course of writing this book, I spoke to couples who had lived with challenging relationships for years. There was the relative with a serious drug addiction who resurfaced routinely looking for money for his latest get-wealthy scheme. The mother so sensitive that she was incensed when she was called by the patient's sister after the patient's surgery instead of the patient's husband. Or the adult child who expected her parents to respond with the same time and energy to her loneliness, even while they themselves struggled with the challenges of chemotherapy.

It can be tempting to try to maintain these relationships as always and pour resources, time, and energy into them—even when those valuable resources are feeling depleted. Normalcy is always tempting: it tells us our lives haven't changed, that we are still capable, and it's a way of proving to ourselves that cancer hasn't robbed us.

The problem is that these relationships may deplete important resources. If we are wasting our energy trying to placate a mother who can't be placated, or draining funds to a drug-abusing brother, then we aren't spending our resources carefully. And worse, these relationships seem to provoke more fighting in couples during the cancer experience than they did prior to a malignancy diagnosis.

For many couples, these relationships have always been a simmering point of tension. When I spoke to Clare Kennedy about her overly sensitive mother, her husband noted that her mother has always been this way and Clare has given more than she should have for years, especially during her illness. His anger was evident when we spoke by phone. He found it difficult to understand why so much time and energy were wasted on a woman so immature. But to Clare, this was still her mother. And placing limits takes energy, too.

That said, there is a clarity that can come to patients during this experience—a new way of seeing relationships and what's truly important. Often this perspective is exactly what we need to make useful changes. Finding a way to express, as gently as possible, that our lives have changed with the onset of cancer and we will no longer be able to do what we've done in the past can be difficult. It can be wrought with complex feelings of guilt and betrayal. But it can also promise intense relief and liberation. And further, there's a satisfaction that comes from feeling that we are capable of changing our lives at a time when cancer has stolen a nip of that vitality.

Some of us have never placed limits on these relationships; we've never said, "No more of this." Or "If you do X, I'm going to do Y, and you won't get what you want anymore." The first time we attempt to do such a thing, we can fear that the world will implode. But from speaking to couples who had made these changes, the result was usually the opposite.

Clare, for instance, eventually did make a change in that she limited her interactions with her mother during crises and stopped believing it was her own responsibility to make her mother feel better.

## 6-3. You may have different views of what's acceptable to tell your friends and family.

I'm a pretty open person and he's pretty private, so sometimes he wishes I'd shut my mouth more. And sometimes I wish he'd open his and share with others.

—ANNA FURGUSON

My husband keeps a journal on CaringBridge and has many "followers" aka fans. . . . There have been times when he would share things I would rather keep private.

—KELLY MOTZ

My husband is a pastor and on a Saturday I told him I didn't want him to talk about my diagnosis. The next morning he started his Sunday sermon by saying, "We have cancer." I was furious.

—RHONDA T.

Some of the worst fights I've seen and heard while writing this book were around privacy. Here's an example of a typical fight. One patient I spoke with had colon cancer, and after her surgery, she briefly required an ostomy bag that collected her body's waste. Her husband shared this detail with friends, and she wanted to beat him around the head and neck.

"What are you thinking?" she asked.

"What?" he replied. "They're our friends."

I want you to understand the benefits and challenges of disclosure so that you'll appreciate both sides of this equation. While I generally have a bias toward encouraging greater disclosure and connection, there are detriments to this as well.

Let's start with the value of connection.

There are some theorists who argue that our culture has overvalued independence and privacy over relationships and connection. Independence as a value has deep roots in our history. Who would have set off across the country in a covered wagon, or worked to farm a plot of land in hostile territory, without a fierce independent streak?

And yet when cancer strikes, we don't get any more points for fighting it alone than we would if we embraced available help. That's right, there's no cosmic scoreboard. But beyond the earliest flood of help from friends, help often doesn't arrive if we don't share what we're going through and open ourselves to the support.

Help can come in a few forms. For many of us, it's helpful just to tell others what's happening. There's a reason why we confess when we've done something wrong, seek support groups when there's anguish in our hearts, and express ourselves through art and writing.

Since the early 1900s, therapists have argued that trying to live silently with painful events is harmful and that talking about these events—even just joking around about them—is beneficial. A growing body of scientific literature supports this and has revealed direct connections between disclosure and health. The first experiments in this area (on college students) found that when participants were asked to write about the "most upsetting experiences of their lives," they went to the health center for illnesses at much lower rates than those students randomly assigned to control groups.[1] More recent studies have found that when they have support, workers are absent from work less, laid-off workers find work faster, and inmates visit the infirmary less; people who have emotional support also demonstrate immediate and lasting immunological benefits involving T-helper cell, natural killer cell, and T-cytotoxic/suppressor cell counts.[2] In a wide range of ill populations—including, for example, those who are HIV positive or have rheumatoid arthritis, chronic fatigue syndrome, or cancer—

groups who express themselves have improvements in health compared with control groups.[3]

Research on women with breast cancer out of Stanford University shows that women who engage and compel others socially have healthier diurnal cortisol slopes than women who routinely push others away (think of cortisol slopes as our daily dose of a buffering stress hormone). In other words, talking about what's in our hearts in a way that compels other people is physically beneficial.

Now let's focus on the benefits of privacy. Privacy is helpful when you are eager to not be treated differently. One of the hard parts of others knowing about your illness—or your spouse's illness—is that you can't control the reaction and the stakes are high. A number of patients shared that they just wanted to be seen as the strong, independent, or funny person they were before the diagnosis, not the "person with cancer that everyone felt sorry for," as one patient phrased it.

Some patients and their spouses shared that keeping things private was especially helpful at work, where concern about losing assigned responsibilities, demotions, or even firing was a realistic possibility. While the Family and Medical Leave Act (FMLA) was designed to protect patients and family members from employment discrimination in larger businesses (those with fifty or more employees) and applies to workers who have worked 1,250 hours, there are many employees who work in smaller businesses or are at new jobs where those protections don't exist. Privacy may be a necessity in circumstances in which disclosure would put a needed job at risk.

And while the FMLA can protect us from losing a job, it can't protect us from losing responsibilities or how we're situated at work. For example, one patient shared that he was in line to lead a new multiyear effort to roll out an expensive product in a four-state territory. He was expected to make decisions about everything from the amount of the product to produce to where and how the product was initially placed with willing distributors.

But soon after he shared his diagnosis, the role was given to a colleague, presumably because his boss wanted assurances that the person in the role would be there for more than one year.

Here's another variable for the soup. For some patients, keeping things private may be possible early in the cancer experience but unrealistic later. That is, our appearance can change radically during some treatments. Those with head and neck cancers, for example, will often have surgeries that are difficult to conceal. Some chemotherapy drugs can shave hair cleaner than a military barber, and there are a number of other side effects of treatments that can betray privacy. In my case, I had rapid weight loss during chemotherapy, swollen prednisone cheeks, baldness, and a greenish pallor. If I were on a bus and you were asked which person on the bus was ill, you'd have picked me out immediately.

When cancer's side effects "out" an otherwise private patient, his or her social supports may know or suspect the patient has cancer before the patient discloses the diagnosis. This often has the paradoxical consequence of the patient getting far *more* attention than they otherwise would have if they had just told everyone—when people start asking one another questions like, "Is Eleanor sick?" or "Did you see her hair coming out during the choral practice?" as happened to one woman I spoke with.

If you are one of those folks who would like to keep your diagnosis (or your spouse's diagnosis) highly private, you should be aware that some people in your network may feel betrayed if they discover the truth. Those individuals may feel they were robbed of an opportunity to be helpful and supportive and that not hearing the diagnosis indicates that you feel they are not a "close enough" friend. Others will suspect you didn't trust them enough. These consequences are paradoxical, because the privacy-seeking individual usually seeks privacy to "keep things the same as they were," but the new information disrupts the old relationship and results in greater distance and even hostility or feelings of hurt.

I want you as a couple to have a practical discussion about the types of help that would be useful to you. Perhaps it's receiving meals; it might be getting rides or having friends with you at chemotherapy or radiation treatments; or it might be just having friends come over to watch movies and *not* talk about cancer.

I also want you to nudge yourself toward telling other people what you are going through. Naturally, there's a balance to find here, but most of us hold too much back and share too little rather than too much.

I have seen too many people starve at a virtual banquet of social support because they believed that they should manage their anguish alone, that talking about the pain in their hearts would reveal weakness, or that no one wanted to hear it.

On the other hand, if you are an individual for whom sharing the diagnosis might have serious negative consequences for your work or social life, I hope you will explain this well enough for your spouse that he or she understands your reasoning, and you can find a negotiated response that will work well enough for both of you.

## 6-4. Don't be afraid of support groups.

So we are both optimistic, and one of the things that helps us get there is education. Learning what we could about this, going to support groups. Meeting people that had dealt with this a lot longer than we had.

—HELEN KELLEY

People are so good. If you push them away you'll miss out on a lot.

—DAVID MILSON

Many of us are wary of spending too much time around other patients, or people who know patients, and some of this fear is reasonable. When I was sick I didn't want to hear stories about people dying, I didn't want to be reminded of what could happen. I didn't want to belong to this group!

The understandable desire to avoid being exposed to bad news can prevent us from getting wisdom from other patients. And there is much wisdom there. In my own case, to put it simply, I would likely not have children if my mother hadn't had the nerve to talk with the mother of another patient. Her son had been through significant treatment, and my mother peppered her with questions. She eventually told my mother about a new urologist in town who had a sperm bank. My mother acted on this information, which our physicians did not share or seem to know about, and the ultimate result is that I now have two adolescents. OK, so maybe this story didn't end as happily as it could have, but they won't be adolescents forever. I hope. And, of course, I'm not suggesting that going to support groups will result in two adolescents living in your house.

Many of the patients I spoke with found great solace as well as helpful information from accepting help from other patients, both informally or through structured support groups. Among other help they received, patients told me, was assistance in dealing with chemotherapy, selecting reconstruction surgeons, finding wigs, negotiating with insurance companies, ideas for maintaining sexuality, and explaining cancer to children.

David Spiegel at Stanford conducted a series of experiments evaluating patients in support groups and found in one cohort that they lived twice as long as people on a waiting list.[4] The survival benefit was not found in replication attempts, but future studies did find that patients who participate in support groups have improved mood and pain relief.[5] We don't have a good understanding of how these groups improve our quality of life, but there's no question that they do.

There's clinical lore among mental health professionals that men tend to like support groups that focus on learning skills and information, while women appear to enjoy groups that are more about relationships, but these stereotypes clearly don't hold for everyone. In addition, it is clear that mixed diagnosis groups can be tough for both the people who are newcomers to the cancer experience and those who are journeymen. In other words, patients with metastatic breast cancer often appear to benefit more from groups with other women who have metastatic disease, rather than mixed groups in which some of the participants will have stage 1 disease. And women with stage 1 disease may struggle in groups with women with more advanced disease.

Support groups offer information, but they also offer us a chance to see our own experiences as they echo in others. Hearing our own words come out of someone else's mouth can be enormously validating and give us an opportunity to gain distance and perspective about our own struggles. For example, one patient told me that he realized he had unrealistic expectations for his wife's recovery when he heard another man express feelings similar to his own in group. There was something about hearing those words come from someone else that gave him the vantage point he needed.

## 6-5. Explore social networking.

The CaringBridge thing has been wonderful. It really has, it's been a great source of getting information out to people and that's probably pumped me up as much as anything, seeing comments. I've had over four thousand hits from people that have responded. People I haven't seen in thirty years, people I coached thirty years ago. The whole spectrum, from the ones I coached last year to people I had their kid in camp back in 1980. Some of the stories are really funny, they perk you up, they take you out of the moment. . . . It gives you a bright spot.

—David Milson

We mostly talk about him, to tell you the truth. I am sick of it. I am sick of that. Every time somebody calls on the phone and they will say, "How is David doing?"

—Barbara Harrison

Very quickly, for those who aren't computer people, social networking typically refers to computer-based communication with other people. Unlike e-mail, social networking provides computer-based environments that make it easy to communicate with a larger network of individuals than individual e-mail might, and these are often supplemented with video, photography, or music.

As we've discussed, of all psychological variables, social support is the most powerful. Whether we are a rat in a cage, a soldier on a battlefield, or a caregiver helping our spouse through gastrointestinal cancer, being supported makes a difference in our wellness.

Social networking Internet sites such as Facebook, Google+, and Twitter are providing survivors and spouses opportunities to connect with one another. Research numbers demonstrate the explosion in the growth of these sites: A study conducted in late 2009 focused on Facebook found that of nearly 300,000 people connected to 757 groups, half or so were for patients and caregivers.[6] Just three years later, the same methodology identified over 600 groups focused on breast cancer alone with a total membership of over 1,000,000![7]

YouTube also offers people the opportunity to make and view video diaries about the illness and caregiving experience, and studies have just started to analyze the videos presented by patients and caregivers online.[8] For individuals looking for specific information, especially about side effects, there is a site called "Patients Like Me," which has stored data from over 120,000 patients across 500 conditions and may be the richest source of accessible data on patient side effects in existence outside of electronic medical records.

CaringBridge is a nonprofit website that offers members the ability to create information-dissemination pages where they can share their stories in a blog format and hear from readers who are likely already in their life. These pages are especially helpful for connecting with individuals slightly outside of the inner social circle, as it allows for acquaintances to hear directly from the patient or caregiver without having to intrude, and then they can communicate back through the pages.

Finding the right fit for us online can be a challenge, but a number of couples I spoke with were using social networking to connect with friends outside of the cancer world or to find likeminded individuals who had also struggled with similar illnesses.

Groups can also assist with information dissemination. Social networking sites can help spouses and patients get information out to everyone in the social network, instead of having to answer the same questions over and over.

## 6-6. It can be very hard to accept the help we need, even when it's offered. That's not a good enough reason to not accept needed help.

I'm trying to let somebody else take care of it because I know when school starts in August I'll have to go back to work. I'll have to allow somebody to come over and do those things for us. I guess it's just letting go of some of the control. I like control. I like everything to be in a line.

—VALREE MILSON

A number of the couples I interviewed said that when they were initially offered assistance from extended family, friends, churchgoers, or coworkers, they rejected it. Many of us have grown up in a society that is firmly rooted in do-it-yourself philosophies. Asking for help, or even receiving help when offered, can feel like failure or something only done by those with no or little pride. But at times, it is too hard to march through the cancer experience without assistance.

Here's the tension point. Some patients want to grind this out without getting help because they are getting what they need from their spouses. But I spoke with a number of spouses who were burning out. They were emotionally and physically exhausted from caretaking, even though they deeply loved the person they were caring for. Simply put, whether they realized it or not, they needed help.

Research indicates that at different times spouses need skill, education, counseling, or help with tasks. When they accept help, caregivers are better able to cope, more confident in their ability to manage stressors, and enjoy a better quality of life.[9]

Taking advantage of help is also usually awkward. It takes energy at first to instruct someone as to what you need, and often people who need help don't get it because they are nurturing the falsehood that it's harder to explain what's needed than to do it oneself.

When I work with a new couple facing cancer, one of the questions I ask early is "What have you done when people have offered to help?" Most couples shrug. To benefit from help, it takes speaking up when a friend or coworker says, "Let me know if we can do anything." The response is usually to say "Thanks" and nothing else. A more productive response would be to say,

"Thank you for the offer. Actually, given how sick Linda has been this week, I'd be very appreciative if you could file those reports for me," or "We've been at the hospital so much, I don't think our plants have been watered. If you could do that for us this week, it would be very helpful. It would just take me a few minutes to explain."

Most people are glad to have something to do to be helpful. It does take some organization to prioritize the things that need to be done.

# 7

# Let's Talk about Sex

In this chapter we turn to the topic of sex. There will be kinky photographs, titillating stories, and fantasies involving whips, pulleys, and a trapeze. OK, maybe not. Instead we'll have some frank conversations about sex during the cancer experience. We'll cover three issues. The first section focuses on the concept of flexibility, because in my experience, most couples are remarkably consistent in their sexual activities and we must often adapt to our new circumstances to stay sexual. Second, I'll speak to those couples for whom sex is no longer physically possible and talk about the need to maintain intimacy even though sex is gone. Finally, some couples stop being sexual because the patient feels deformed or unattractive. These individuals forget how adaptable the human sexual response truly is.

## 7-1. Though we may not be able to be sexual in the exact same way we once were, most couples can still be fabulously sexual.

I just have no desire. It's hard to talk to him about it, because you know, he just thinks it's him. And it's not him! I try to tell him all the time it's not him. It's just my body. It's hard for him not to feel rejected.

—DIANA KOUNK

The biggest change is she's way more tired now. . . . It's not even something that crosses my mind now because I know she can't handle it physically.

—TOBIN HODGES

My husband had to have his gall bladder out by the same doctor that did my surgery. And he came home from the hospital—they don't keep you long—and I think I had just had my stitches out from my breast cancer surgery the day before. . . . So he comes home and we are in bed and my doctor had said to us, "You can resume your sex life whenever you want to," and ha ha, I just turned around and said that to my husband and we had to laugh because we were both feeling so terrible.

—BARBARA JANZEN

The research shows that about half of all women treated for cancers of the reproductive organs[1] and half of men treated for prostate cancer[2] have long-term sexual challenges. Virtually every couple I spoke with had some sexual changes associated with cancer. But a great number also rediscovered, or in some cases reinvented, their sexuality.

Forgive me a brief digression. When I was in graduate school we were required to enroll in a variety of psychology courses that weren't closely related to clinical work. Many were dull. One of the most notorious for boredom was titled "Comparative Psychology," which actually meant ethology, or animal behavior. It didn't help that the professor's voice sounded like an air conditioner with a broken fan belt. *Yawn.*

At one point the professor taught us about the stickleback fish, a little silvery fellow found in freshwater in Europe, Asia, and North America. The professor was actually trying to teach us about issues with decision-making (stickleback fish make better decisions when they are in large groups) but also took a few moments to describe the sexual behavior of the fish. Given the tedium in the room, I perked up when he mentioned sex. Even fish sex.

The little stickleback fish turns out to be remarkably consistent. When they mate, they do a fancy little fish dance, in the same order. The male swims in a zig-zag pattern (hey, baby); the female turns her nose up and swims toward the nest. He puts his little snout in the entrance. She follows. He prods her tail. And then . . .

Sorry. The next part is censored. Let's leave the little sticklebacks just a moment of privacy, shall we?

This is what caught my attention. Imagine being able to reliably predict what a fish is going to do next! Where it's going to swim! What it's going to do with its little fish nose! It's incredible.

Then, later in graduate school and as a clinician, I learned about human sexuality, which is considerably more varied. *Except that sometimes it isn't.* Clearly, there is wide variation in how couples have sex—including when, what, where, and how. But after talking to patients for twenty years about their sex lives, I can tell you that inside a given couple's repertoire of sexual behavior, things are often very consistent from one encounter to the next. That's right. Many of us are just like those bastions of watery consistency—the little stickleback fish.

For example, most couples can tell me which partner is the one who always initiates (there are many couples who share initiation, but far more who have the same person initiate) and the code for "let's have sex." Here are a few of the codes for "let's have sex":

*She turns off the lamp on my side of the bed.*

*He says, "Let's get busy."*

*She says, "Are you feeling it?"*

*She just grabs me. You know. There.*

*He puts on music.*

And my favorite: *She hums the theme music to the movie* Jaws.

What happens next is also usually consistent. Over time couples learn how they physically fit together best—the position where things are the most exciting—or both members feel the best emotionally, and couples typically have a limited repertoire of familiar behaviors. And then they do the same thing again and again until one of them decides that *this time, we're doing something different.*

For many couples, this works well for years, until cancer strikes. It is a cosmic interruption of healthy sex.

And in the midst of the cancer experience, there are many reasons why sex doesn't happen. First, above all, most couples simply don't talk about sex. Most of the couples I interviewed had sexual changes during cancer. For some couples, cancer literally changed the plumbing; for others, his or her cancer was fed by hormones like estrogen or testosterone that are tightly related to sexual function. And still others are just too emotionally spent to muster any energy for humming the music to *Jaws*.

Cancer can render us bald and swollen, and change how our bodies look. Psychologically, these changes can result in the patient feeling profoundly unattractive and worry that he or she has "lost it." We may also have fresh scars, or be missing key appendages like breasts that once occupied considerable sexual energy. Even if we can have intercourse, cancer can interrupt key parts of the experience. Forty percent of men who have radical prostatectomies, for example, note that they can't have orgasms or that their orgasms are considerably less powerful.[3]

On the other side, the partner often feels that they shouldn't force the patient to have sex when they are feeling ill or otherwise infirm. So if both people want to have sex but both are nervous about pressuring the other person or feeling that they aren't sexy anymore, sex may not happen. Poor fishies.

While many of us view sex as a stress-reliever, the truth appears to be that sex is more like the proverbial canary in the coal mine. Research shows that, for most couples, it's the first thing to go when there's intense stress.

It is unfortunate—but true—that cancer may force couples who have never spoken about sex to talk about it. From the patient side, when we're ready, we have to tell our partners that we still want to have sex. This is key. And even if the plumbing has changed dramatically—rendering intercourse impossible, for example—it is still possible to be terrifically sexual.

Couples I spoke with who couldn't have intercourse anymore had evolved some clever ways of coping. One couple took turns masturbating while the other talked dirty to them. Another couple gave long massages to each other and then used oral sex and vibrators to accomplish what they could not otherwise. Still another reduced their focus on orgasms and turned instead to long sensual oil massages.

By the way, it's worth mentioning that for breast cancer patients, the type of surgery a woman has (from minor lumpectomy to double mastectomy) does not impact long-term self-image or sexual functioning. Instead it looks like women's self-esteem and sexuality going into the cancer experience are a better predictor of sexuality long-term.[4] Let me say that again. It's not the extensiveness of the surgery that impacts sexuality for women who have breast cancer.

An issue that came up for a few couples I spoke with (no pun intended) was how difficult it is to adjust to new ways of functioning sexually while simultaneously missing the ways we used to be. One woman, Helen Kelley, whose husband had prostate surgery that severed the nerves that made spontaneous erections possible, shared this with me: "He doesn't have sexual function without outside help. He managed to do what he needed to do—he took shots—to have an erection but he couldn't seem to overcome the parts in his head that said he should be able to do this on his own. I got so angry with him. . . .

He was so caught up in that that he couldn't enjoy the moment of us being together."

Then later, when she developed breast cancer herself and needed to have surgeries, she softened: "Maybe we all go through that a little bit, thinking of it going back the way it used to be."

Helen Kelley's is an important observation. Men's loss of sexual potency is profoundly psychologically challenging for them, with over three-quarters reporting a loss of sexual identity and half feeling reduced self-esteem if they cannot produce erections following surgery.[5] For those who haven't experienced this, it might seem absurd. *It wasn't his fault, he still seems virile and manly to me* . . . But for men, impotency is associated with being terribly aged and emasculated.

The willingness to talk, and flexibility to reimagine sexuality, is the most important characteristic held in common by the couples who continued having sex. As many sex experts have noted, the most important sexual organ we have is our brains.

Just in case you think you are too old for sex, let's review a recent study published in the *New England Journal of Medicine*, the most prestigious medical journal in the United States. After lengthy interviews with over three thousand Americans between the ages of fifty-seven and eighty-five, the lead author, Stacy Tessler-Lindau, concluded that most Americans are sexually active well through their sixties and that more than half of the people interviewed had sex well into their eighties. Incidentally, half also described some sexual problems, including diminished desire, vaginal dryness, or erectile difficulties, but only one-third of men, and only one-fifth of women, ever discussed these issues with physicians.[6]

So, talk to your partner and let them know that you're still interested or willing to try. Be creative. Be flexible. Stay engaged. Let your partner know that you are still attracted. If you do these things, there's a very good chance a healthy sex life will return, even if it isn't exactly the same as before.

## 7-2. Some couples are physically unable to have sex. That's a loss. But intimacy and sex are not the same. Don't lose intimacy, too.

I have no function whatsoever as a man would, but I agreed to do that to save my life. . . . Certainly sex is a good thing to have if you are able, but if you are not able, there is intimacy. There is love and compassion. There is a lot more to an existence with a spouse than just having physical sex.

—DAVID HARRISON

Sex is only as important as you make it. That's the way I look at it. . . . I'd rather him be well and be here.

—BARBARA HARRISON

A handful of couples I spoke with are unable to have intercourse and that function will likely never return. In a few cases, men had prostate surgeries that eliminated their ability to produce an erection. One of the men I spoke with was offered a penile implant by his physician, but the couple talked about it and he declined, feeling that another surgery (on top of the many he'd already endured) was not worth the added risk.

There's no question that losing sexuality is a profound loss for some. In fact, of all of the topics I spoke about with couples, their sexuality and feelings about sexuality produced the greatest variation. Some individuals were deeply saddened and even angry that they had lost their ability to have sex. But others simply moved on, choosing to focus instead on living.

Couples I spoke with who would likely never have intercourse again told me that they needed to adjust and encourage other types of intimacy. They had started having more meals together, walking together, and going to movies. I'd expected that they'd compensate with other types of touch, but the opposite was the case for a few couples. "Touching just reminds us of what we can't do anymore, so we hug and hold hands but that's where it usually ends," one woman shared. Others increased their casual, nonsexual touch, like when they passed in the hallway or were near one another in the kitchen.

Barbara Harrison shared that the most unusual response to losing intercourse came from one of her friends. A friend of hers joked, "All the girls here are so jealous of you" because she didn't have to deal with being pressured by men anymore. "They said you are so lucky that you don't have to deal with this at sixty-five."

## 7-3. If you haven't asked your spouse, you're just guessing how your lover will view your new body.

We'll get into this topic with a story.

It's a handful of weeks after my wife's double mastectomy surgery. Both breasts are gone and she's had "expanders" put in so that she can pursue reconstruction later.

When I arrive home from work Terry is in front of the television wrapped in a blanket, watching *American Drivel* reruns. I see her a little later emptying the dishwasher and then she's outside sweeping in front and now she's . . . I don't know.

Right now, my daughter is looking for my wife. The seven-year-old has a school project to complete involving glitter, glue, and small mirrors. Oh, and a potato. Somehow these objects have something to do with a book titled *Nim's Island*.

I check outside in the back and the front, and then in the garage. She isn't in our bedroom or the girls'. She isn't with Abby, who is napping in the playroom beneath her favorite blanket. Nor is she with the dog, perched, as usual, on the hot-tub cover. The minivan is still in the garage. Hmmm. I'm making a circle back through our bedroom when I hear something in our walk-in closet.

I open the door, and the crack of light finds a blue thigh.

She's on her knees on the carpet, surrounded by hanging slacks and shoes. She wears only her blue sweatpants, her hands are over her face and her elbows cover her naked torso. The bandages that had been wrapped tightly around her chest are snaked around her ankles; in the dim light from the hallway they look like sailor's rope.

"Please don't turn on the light," she says. Her voice is taut and gasping.

"Mom?" Alex is suddenly behind me.

"Not now, honey. I'll be out in a sec," Terry says. She says it with a voice I have yet learned to master. It carries absolute maternal certainty, and Alex withdraws silently.

"What's going on? Alex was looking for you. I think she wants help with her . . ."

"*Nim's Island,*" Terry says.

"Funniest thing, she has this potato . . ."

There's a pause, and then Terry doubles over onto her knees and emits a wailing sob. It's a pure silver tone, anguished and grating and it slices away all the humor in the universe.

She lets her hands drop to her sides and slowly comes up; her torso is in the light and my eyes have adjusted. There are modest bulbs where her breasts used to be. No nipples yet.

"You're going to leave me," she says.

What?!

"No. Look at me," she orders. "This is who I am now," she says. She pulls off her baseball cap and there's one lone strand of hair left.

I'm startled. I don't want to be, but I am. It's true that her chest looks bizarre. As if finding a craggy parking lot where my childhood home once stood. It's familiar but not. There are black, crimson stitches and a port, where the cosmetic surgeon can access her breasts to inflate them with more saline. And without eyebrows her face lacks its usual brightness, not to mention her bald head.

"You're going to leave," she says again.

"That's ridiculous," I say. But I'm still standing and I sound more like a professor than a husband, so I drop and sit on my knees at her level and now I'm more like a husband and see, down here, we're in this together, only my words don't match my new position. And suddenly I remember looking at breasts on the Internet last night and we haven't had sex and why am I thinking about this now?

But I launch into a reasoned and loving explanation that who she is hasn't changed and I remember feeling vulnerable when I had cancer and she stayed with me and then I wrap up with a few nicely chosen words about the children and our lives together and even Bisbee the dog and it's a diatribe but it's not horrible. Is it?

One corner of her mouth is turned up. She's studying me carefully and seems disappointed. She could have delivered this speech herself, it's too canned. But I don't know what else to say so I just stand up, getting tougher now.

"Come on. You have to get up. Put on a shirt. *Nim's Island* is waiting and apparently everyone in this house knows I can't carve a potato into a magical creature." This, apparently, does strike a chord, if only a minor one, and now she wipes her face, rises to standing, and yells "I'm coming" to Alex across the house.

Men do not routinely leave their wives when they have cancer. In a series of studies, researchers in Quebec interviewed women with breast cancer three months, eighteen months, and then eight years after the women's diagnoses.[7] The interviews focused on their relationships. The same researchers used cold calls to find other couples in the same age groups and conducted interviews with them, too. Marriages in which cancer had visited did not break down any more often than other marriages. But low marital satisfaction just three months after diagnosis was predictive of problems later.

The same research group then decided to investigate if relationships in which the man has prostate cancer are any different from breast cancer couples. First, they found, of course, that the couples with prostate cancer are older. In many cases they'd been together twenty years longer. But there was other news, too. The men with prostate cancer reported feeling better understood by their wives than women with breast cancer reported feeling understood by husbands. Message received.

It's true that I was shocked by my wife's appearance. But I had no thoughts about leaving. Just like I wouldn't cut off my own arm if it was disfigured. But I didn't know how to convince her of this.

Many people I've interacted with who have to undergo transformative procedures on their faces, breasts, or lower regions often harbor the suspicion that their spouse is going to abandon them. These fears seem to surface even when couples have been together successfully for a long time. The problem in many of these situations is that couples don't speak.

It need not be much of a conversation, but I strongly recommend that spouses share their thoughts with their husbands and wives out loud. A few encouraging words can make an enormous difference. JoAnn McClure, one woman I interviewed, put it well, and she should know. JoAnn had breast cancer twice and underwent a mastectomy. Then, years later, she had colon cancer and had to have her rectum removed. She shared that it takes time to adjust to each new physical reality, but eventually, "You get used to it. It's something you have to do, you don't have an option."

# 8

# Closeness and Making Peace with Dependence

Cancer can be a cosmic wake-up call that restructures how we think about our time. The first part of this chapter focuses on allowing cancer to clarify how we spend time together. Then I turn to a few predictable closeness killers, including bickering, which, while common, can be destructive, even when we are used to it.

In the latter part of the chapter I address common struggles with navigating dependence. Being dependent is painful. Some patients respond by pushing away the people they most need. I've also seen some patients rely so much on others that when they are more capable, they have difficulty exerting independence again. We'll illuminate these challenges, and I give spouses some direct advice to help patients rediscover independence when necessary.

# 8-1. Allow cancer to clarify how you spend your time with one another.

I am going to have plenty of time to cry later. Right now I want to enjoy our being together and having the time that we do and being able to think about things in more depth.

—JODY PRICE

You will fall apart if you don't keep going. . . . There are many people that just hover in the house and don't go anywhere or do anything. They stop living. We had tickets to the Lakeland center and I went with my walker and I think once I even went in the wheelchair. You have to keep going or you get moldy.

—JOANN MCCLURE

The first thing we did right after treatment, we signed up with a group called "Tempest Tours." These are guys that are the best storm chasers in the country so we signed on with them. They took us out in a van. . . . Sometimes we would drive six hours to see a really good storm.

—NANCY N.

While writing this book I met couples who raided their "rainy day fund" to pay for a housekeeper and someone to mow the lawn so that they could focus on what they wanted to do instead of housework. Others learned to ski and planned a cruise; I heard about bird-watching trips, storm chasing, and sports fans who finally went to live games.

Cancer does not automatically recenter our perspectives.

Many couples march through the experience without any change in how they spend time. Yet, having something fun to look forward to as a couple can make treatment just a little easier.

Nancy N. and her husband decided that chasing storms was the thing for them. They'd always been curious about this mix of science and danger, so as soon as treatment was over they scoured the Internet for a professional group who got close to tornadoes, severe thunderstorms, and my favorite, flash floods (if you're curious, Tempest Tours has advice on their Web site for how to handle flash floods). Then they did it.

During my bone marrow transplant I decided I wanted to learn how to scuba dive, and as soon as I was well enough, we took lessons and got certified in the cool, crystal clear waters of Ginnie Springs along the banks of the Santa Fe River in Northern Florida.

It doesn't have to be a "bucket list" activity to be enjoyable. Some couples just changed how they spent time—having more conversations about things they enjoyed. Even trips to treatment can offer opportunities to reconnect, given the hectic pace of some lives. David Milson, for example, was treated in a few cancer centers in Texas. He and his wife had to travel back and forth to Houston from where they lived four hours away. "It was actually a lot of quality time," he told me. "We hadn't had that kind of time together in twenty years, since we had kids. I think it was really good."

# 8-2. Turn off the bickering.

He stopped picking at me. We've been married thirty-two years, you know the things that I don't do right, that I've never done right? The same things that he doesn't do right, that he's never done right. These are never going to change. During those early months everything I did was OK. I didn't get yelled at if I didn't remember to write a little slip into the checkbook if I used the debit card or something.

—Diana Kounk

He says, "Stop yelling at me." I say, "I am not yelling. That is my voice, I can't help it."

—Barbara Harrison

My wife changes the thermostat without telling me. She'd be comfortable if it was warm enough to roast chickens. Seriously, there are times in the bedroom when I expect a bunch of older naked Turkish men with towels to waddle by and sit in the sauna we call a bedroom.

She uses her phone as an alarm in the mornings and sets it to go off three times, often forgetting it's still set after she's up and having breakfast—while I'm still in bed. She hangs her longest dresses over my shoe tree so that I can't find my shoes.

I know, horrible crimes right? And shouldn't I remind her—implore, cajole, argue, point, and flail—at every opportunity when she subjects me to these indignities?

*Sigh.*

OK, perhaps it's true that occasionally—well, most of the time—I leave my socks on the floor where I've taken them off. I forget to spray down the shower door with the special spray bottle she bought to avoid staining. I watch television with the speakers blaring. My side of the bed is often like a nest with a pile of novels I think I'm reading, newspapers, consumer magazines, photography books, and whatever found its way into my pockets. For some odd reason she thinks it's reasonable to point out these foibles, when clearly they aren't a big deal.

We've been married more than twenty years and this list isn't much different than it was ten or fifteen years ago. We could substitute out a few things for a few new things, but mostly, it's the same stuff. Clearly, pointing these issues out to each other isn't effective, and yet we did it routinely.

When breast cancer struck we took a break from reminding each other of our various crimes. And given how effective the reminders were—i.e., *not at all*—this was not a bad thing.

Pick your metaphor: With our spouse, when cancer visits, it's OK to be more of a fan than a coach. A diner instead of a food critic. An audience member instead of the director. We can do more applauding and less criticizing.

Here's another way to think of this. Imagine a dark sky and a tiny lifeboat in the middle of the ocean. We can just discern two little people on board as we get closer. The waves are high, and at any moment the boat threatens to capsize, sending its occupants into the salty froth. Up goes the boat, down goes the boat. On board the two little people clutch for purchase to avoid the freezing waters.

Now let's get closer where we can hear what they are shouting, over the sound of the waves.

"But you always leave your socks on the floor? Who am I, your maid?"

"Can't you turn off your damned alarm after it goes off once and you get up?"

"Oh yeah? Are you so brain-damaged that you can't squeegee down the shower door after your shower?"

"At least I can sleep in a temperature range below those required by lizards, snakes, and fire coral."

As I've written, I'm not grateful to have had cancer. I'm not grateful that Terry had cancer. But I was not given a choice. And there are these rare bits of life wisdom. One of them, perhaps the most important of them, was this one.

When Terry was diagnosed I finally saw those little foibles for what they truly were. Her quirky, unique way of navigating this odd planet. That they occasionally irritated me was no more meaningful than the fact that I don't always like the weather. And they are never going to change. But with them comes this incredible woman.

## 8-3. For many, being at peace with dependence takes hard work.

Who's going to be here for him in the way he's been here for me? I can't pay it back. I'm going to die first.

—Ann Shapiro

I found dependence startling.

Here I was, this twenty-two-year-old man accustomed to hopping in the shower, grabbing a bagel, and rushing from my dorm room—hair still wet—a bag of books in a canvas knapsack.

But hospitalized in the midst of a bone marrow transplant, every move had to be planned. First, I'll swing my legs off the bed, careful not to catch the IV running into my central line on the bedrails. Then I'll get on my slippers because the floor is freezing. Then I'll push the IV pole around the wall-mounted television and into the bathroom. I'll turn on the water and sit, waiting for it to get warm enough. If I get dizzy, I'll wait for Terry. Hmmm. Maybe I should have Terry start the hot water before I get out of bed. That means asking her to help me. Screw that. I can do this on my own.

She comes into the room as I'm trying to navigate the IV pole around the television mounted high on the wall, but I've gotten the IV line caught on the power cord, which I should have anticipated, but I'm out of position to reach up and pull it down and I'm worried that if I put too much tension on it, I might yank it out of my body—which would be a cosmic bummer. Gravity has been turned up. I feel exhausted. But I want to do this myself.

Terry stares at me as if I've just decided to drink motor oil. "What are you doing?"

"Nothing. Leave me alone," I snap. Her eyebrows lift and she takes a step back. OK, cowboy, she seems to be saying with her eyes, if you're such a big man, let's see how you navigate this without help. Of course, I actually do need help and we both know it. The IV line is trapped over the television cord and unless I suddenly grow a new appendage like a science-fiction squid, I'm stuck. But I don't admit it nearly soon enough, because I'm stubborn and there's a little voice inside me demanding that I do this myself.

After I tug on the IV line a few times, I shrug, defeated. I give up. I'm an idiot. Terry gracefully steps forward and quickly releases my leash, and I'm into the bathroom without so much as thanking her.

We have a choice about how we respond to being dependent. We can be angry, resigned, avoidant, or resentful. Or, we can be appreciative. Grateful. Encouraging. I admit that I wrestled between these poles more than I should have. I could have made life easier for Terry and my friends if I'd simply been more grateful and less stubborn.

## 8-4. If you feel guilty because your spouse is taking care of you, don't take it out on them!

You've been a guy that's done everything forever and now all of a sudden you can't get up, go to the bathroom. There's been a huge amount of guilt 'cause I want to get up, I really want to get up. You want to do those—you want to take care of yourself and you don't want to burden them. I've got a daughter that's going to be a sophomore in high school. I don't want to take anything away from her summer and my wife. It's like everything is revolving around me and it shouldn't be.

—DAVID MILSON

A handful of patients shared with me, usually after a considerable interview, that they felt guilty that their partner had to take care of them. This may seem surprising to folks who haven't witnessed this relationship pattern for themselves. But for those of us who have always been fiercely independent, capable, and strong, the new dependence that occasionally comes packaged with cancer can be a terrible blow.

We may need help with everything. At one point or another

during my five-year trajectory with cancer, I needed assistance with walking, opening doors, getting down from scanner tables, preparing food, shopping, showering, and, as my memory vacillated with treatment, remembering names, regimen, phone numbers, and even my bank card pin number.

While recovering from heavy chemotherapy, I behaved like an elderly man. Given that I was only twenty-five years old, this was a bizarre and new experience. It was also emotionally challenging.

Dependence is enormously difficult for some of us. It can feel like we're a burden, dragging down the people around us. The qualities that initially made us attractive to our spouses—our strength or capabilities—may feel like a distant memory.

Yet, we can't—should not—ever—do you hear me? Never ever take it out on them.

Here's the hard truth: Some of us push other people away when we feel like a burden. Almost like elephants who go off to die alone, we antagonize the people we love in a twisted effort to protect them. The horrible logic goes like this: *If they stop taking care of me then they will be happier. If I can tick them off enough, they'll go away and be better off.* Of course on the spouse side, they end up feeling punished even though they've been doing the best they can. And only rarely does the pushing away work. Usually the spouse stays, and just mutters to him- or herself, "I'm doing all this terrific work to help him or her and this is the reward I get?!"

And this is the type of thing the spouse usually can't talk about with anyone else. No one wants to say, "Yeah, my husband is going through chemotherapy—and he's been such pond scum about the whole thing!"

When I was the spouse during Terry's breast cancer experience, I was happy to help. I love her, and liked feeling that I could do something to fight back against the cancer. In return, I just wanted her praise. I wanted her to appreciate the work I was doing, even if it was mediocre sometimes. I wanted to hear, "Wow, nice job, didn't know you had it in you!" or just a simple "Thanks."

Spouses sometimes respond with deep doubts about themselves. "Is she pushing me away because she wishes she had someone else to take care of her?" "Is he being such a tool because he'd be happier without me?" "Am I not helping in the right ways?"

It's OK to say, "I hate being dependent" or "I hate relying on you." Or perhaps, "I wish I wasn't such a burden." Even better, try, "Wow, you are doing an amazing job taking care of me."

## 8-5. There is such a thing as too much dependence. If you're the spouse, if you don't absolutely need to do everything for your lover who has cancer, don't. They should still be taking care of themselves, too.

It can be a little uncomfortable to balance.

—JODY PRICE

Of all the complex situations we face, perhaps one of the most challenging is moving between dependence and independence. Consider Jack, who was married to Preeti for fifteen years. A patient with early pancreatic cancer, Jack had a pancreaticoduodenectomy, the most common operation to remove cancer of the exocrine pancreas. The surgery removed the "head" of the pancreas and part of the body of the organ. Surgeons also removed part of his small intestine and stomach as well as a number of lymph nodes. Following this aggressive surgery he had infections, bleeding, and his stomach often failed to empty itself, leading to pain and discomfort.

Those initial months following his procedure were tough. He was in and out of bed, and tried a variety of diets to improve his stomach function. Preeti, a real-estate attorney, severely limited her practice to take care of Jack. She researched diets and started to manage Jack's insulin, a necessity now that he'd lost a portion of his pancreas. His energy waned and he relied on her for most things outside of the bathroom. Food, company, and the management of his medication.

But even four months after surgery, Jack showed little improvement. By then they'd found a diet that worked (low-fat chicken, fish, eggs) and his insulin was stabilized. But Jack was still relying on Preeti for everything. Her practice was still only hobbling along, and she was afraid to leave his side because every time she did, his pain seemed to return.

It was time for Jack to start exerting more independence. Unfortunately, it took outside intervention in the form of his sister, who visited from out of state and was startled to see her once-boisterous brother so sedate and dependent. But after observing them for a few days she physically yet playfully restrained Preeti from running to the kitchen every time Jack made a request from the couch. "If he can walk to the bathroom, he can walk to the kitchen!" she demanded. "I promise, Jack won't starve out there."

It was true.

It took some work in therapy for the couple to unravel the intense level of dependence Jack had developed on Preeti, but with some ground rules established, Jack was able to crawl back to caring for himself, and Preeti was able to return to working her normal hours, though they had some conflicts during the transition. In treatment we recalibrated their expectations about routines. Jack would take over giving himself his insulin and monitoring his blood sugars. He would share the cooking as he had prior to getting sick. He would start exercising. He would not call for Preeti to deliver him food and reading materials if he was capable of getting them himself.

Preeti and Jack's story is not unusual. It can be scary for both members of a couple to break dependent patterns after they've been established; yet if they last longer than needed, these can be destructive because they freeze the couple at lower function than is possible. Jack wasn't getting out of the house or exercising, and Preeti's practice was suffering.

The first bits of independence are usually hardest to initiate. Jack was initially reticent to manage his insulin by himself and listed a number of reasons, none especially persuasive, why he couldn't do it. In my office, Preeti, soft-spoken and gentle, ran her fingers along his arm and looked away from him, saying, "No, you can do this, I think." He was going to continue his resistance, but she turned suddenly toward him, her face like a mother's, and he quieted.

Preeti's nonjudgmental encouragement was critical in Jack's gaining confidence to take over self-care. This is the take-home message. A firm but encouraging approach by the spouse is essential. You can do this.

In psychological terms, our judgments about our abilities to do a specific thing are called "self-efficacy." Albert Bandura is the father of the study of self-efficacy and he found that once self-efficacy for one activity is initiated, it tends to generalize to other situations. And as Albert would have predicted, once Jack began taking care of his insulin himself, he also began to do other activities he'd stopped, like driving and grocery shopping.

# 9

# Navigating Our Relationship at the End of Life

The first lesson in this chapter is for everyone. I'm going to challenge you to complete an advanced directive that dictates what you want done medically if you are no longer able to speak for yourself. I think all couples should complete these, ideally, in front of each other so your wishes are clear. I'll share a true story I learned while researching this book that powerfully illustrates the need.

The next two sections are addressed to patients and spouses facing the end of life. If you aren't facing end-of-life issues, you might want to skip this section. We'll talk about key issues to consider at the end of life and how to communicate with staff about these. Finally, I'll talk about grief.

# 9-1. Have the "what if?" conversation and complete advanced directives.

My first advice to any couple would be find out what your partner wants in case of needing to make the decision to put someone on life support.

—Penny Carruth

There was something in me that felt like if I wrote it down, I would be inviting it.

—Diana Kounk

I'm going to live to be an old man.

—Harman Spence

You ARE an old man.

—Linda Spence

When I phoned Mel Carruth, a strapping man from a rural area outside of Dallas, he was closing the pawnshop for the night. His voice was strong and he asked if it would be OK if we spoke while he drove home. He mentioned in our conversation that he and his wife had had a tough few years with his lymphoma, and that he'd even been coded a few times. But he didn't remember much about that period. He especially didn't remember one very difficult night.

Later, Penny, his wife of more than twenty years, shared the details. Mel had been struggling with his breathing, so they'd rushed to the emergency room. A steady stream of health professionals came to see him and eventually told them that Mel's situation was quite serious. They tried a variety of quick-acting treatments, like inhalers and giving him adrenaline, but none seemed to improve Mel's breathing. And in addition to his being dehydrated, a variety of his lab values were grim.

Finally, a pulmonologist told Penny that Mel needed to be in the intensive care unit upstairs where they could ensure he was getting enough oxygen. She assented. Mel was whisked away to the elevators while Penny climbed the stairs. When she arrived, she was given a form by one of the professionals.

Here's how she described what happened next. "I signed for him to go on a ventilator. We had never discussed it. Mel is claustrophobic. . . . They put a mask on his face and he fought it and fought it. They got his hands restrained." She paused, and then said, "Watching him all night long jerking and fighting with the mask. It got to the point they had to intubate him with the tube down his throat. It was the longest night of my life, and I was thinking, 'Have I made the right decision?'"

Penny is not alone.

There are roughly 2.4 million deaths in the United States every year,[1] and 70 percent[2] of us are not thinking clearly in our last days when decisions need to be made, leaving our loved ones to make decisions for us. As Penny's situation attests, these are frequently difficult situations. In one study, four out of five caregivers who had to make surrogate decisions had symptoms of post-traumatic stress disorder.[3]

Terry and I have been around medical environments for a long time. We've seen great variation in how physicians communicate during these challenging times. The reality is that it's impossible to know as a patient or spouse whether a transfer onto a ventilator is likely to be temporary or permanent. Research shows that the vast majority of us don't want our last moments to be on a ventilator.

Before we get to that situation, we need to have these conversations. The easiest way to have the conversation, according to experts Drs. Benjamin Levi and Michael Green at Penn State, is to find a good advanced directive and then complete them *together—one for each of us.* By that I mean that the patient describes what he or she wants while the partner asks questions and writes down the answers. In this way, we can assure that both partners are on the same page.

The National Cancer Institute has fact sheets and resources online that can assist individuals in completing and understanding how advanced directives work.

Here's one way to think about it. Advanced directives are a lasting gift we can and should give our families.

## 9-2. At the end of life, communicate with spouses and physicians and nurses about what you want.

We did not have the time that I would have liked to have been able to spend. The chemo and the radiation—when they knew it was that close—I wish it had never been done because that would have given us a couple extra months of quality time. We never really had any. Take the two months if they are going to give you more radiation and chemo and enjoy yourself instead. We missed that.

—Peggy Langdon

We've had some conflicts, for a while it was about him continuing treatment. I wasn't going to be OK with it, but after this last time I think he realized it was not a good thing.

—JODY PRICE

This lesson is about the end of life. It's not for everyone, so if you don't need to think about this now, move along to another lesson, there's nothing to see here. This *is* for those who have found that numerous treatments have stopped working, or are no longer working, and are wondering how to navigate the future so that they are not suffering and can avoid burdening loved ones.

Let's face it, the end of life is not an easy phase and the stakes are high. Doctors may not talk about this, but we need to. I spoke to a number of patients' spouses who had regrets about how their loved one had been treated, medically, at the end of life. In almost all cases, the patient had been treated more aggressively than the spouse wished they had been. Patients had ingested more chemotherapy than they wanted, had life-saving treatments attempted more often than they'd desired, and been in hospitals instead of home more often than they wanted.

Here's the ugly problem. Many oncologists will treat us aggressively right up until the end. It's true that in some cases, chemotherapy and radiation can make us more comfortable when our cancers are incurable. For example, these treatments can sometimes shrink tumors that cause discomfort and relieve bone pain. But in many cases, chemotherapy also causes burdensome side effects. For couples at the end of life hoping to enjoy one another's company until the end, one of the most profound problems is the assault to our thinking caused by chemotherapy.

These are very difficult discussions to have with cancer doctors, who vary in how skilled they are in having direct conversations at the end of life. And it can be very difficult for a spouse to raise the issue if the patient appears to want to continue having treatment. In general, physicians have gotten much better at discussing end-of-life care, but they still tend to wait until the very last minute to bring up the topic, when reducing treatment aggressiveness is no longer possible. It's also worth noting that end-of-life conversations are strongly influenced by the culture of the patient and the physician. Black patients, for example, are far more likely to receive aggressive end-of-life care (when they don't want it) than white patients.[4]

One challenging dynamic occurs when the patient wants to be brave for his or her family, and not allow anyone to "give up hope." He or she can demand ongoing treatment even when all medical information available suggests that the treatment is futile. Cancer doctors sometimes play unwitting accomplices by not having direct conversations at the end of life. When a spouse is less enamored of the idea of the brave patient but would rather have quality time, they can feel afraid to challenge the prevailing plan. No one wants to be the one telling a doctor to stop treatment when the doctor and the patient appear to agree on the right course.

In these circumstances, I suggest asking the hard questions. Such as, "Do you feel this treatment is likely to extend my wife or husband's life or improve his or her quality of life? Should we consider stopping treatment? I want us to enjoy each other and avoid hospitalizations at this stage. What's the best way to accomplish this?" or, "Do you believe we have done everything we reasonably could have to cure this disease?"

Here's a secret. Physicians are not very accurate at telling us how long we are going to live. Dr. Nicholas Christakis at Harvard and his colleagues looked at studies that asked physicians to predict how long a patient was going to live, and then compared those predictions with how long those patients really lived. Physicians were generally accurate when death was within four weeks, but as they make longer estimates they were poorer at estimating, and, notably, they usually overestimated.[5] Which stinks.

In fact, in Dr. Christakis's study, 63 percent of physicians overestimated survival time. It's especially interesting that the more a physician cares about us, the worse they estimate in our favor. The danger with long estimates is that they can rob us of a chance to say, "Thank you, I love you, and don't forget to water the plants."

In all seriousness, some of those conversations are very important. In her last months, my mother told my father and me that she wanted him to have relationships after she was gone. "I don't want him to be alone," she said, and then she pointed a finger at me. "And you can be supportive." If my mother hadn't had those important conversations, I think our lives after would have been much harder. I would have felt more ambivalent when he started dating again, and he might have avoided new relationships.

It's easy to get angry at physicians for not being accurate in their predictions, but these conversations are incredibly difficult. Most physicians want to be optimistic, and as the physician and surgeon Atul Gawande has written, most doctors worry far more about being pessimistic than about being optimistic. "Doctors are especially hesitant to trample on a patient's expectations. . . . And talking about dying is enormously fraught. . . . The last thing you want to do is grapple with the truth."[6] In integrative medicine, a growing movement nationally, physicians are routinely lambasted for "hexing" their patients by giving them too much bad news; so many physicians avoid painting a bleak picture, even when not being completely truthful has drawbacks, too.

And if we haven't taken the time to articulate how we want to pass into the great beyond, and we end up in a hospital, decisions will be made to lengthen our lives as much as possible, even if this only means extending an uncomfortable dying process, or worse.

The other option is to be clear about what we want with our spouses and our physicians. In medical language, this means requesting palliative or hospice care. We can be referred to hospice when, in a physician's opinion, the natural trajectory of our illness will take our lives within six months. (It doesn't actually have to take our lives that quickly for hospice to be continually reimbursed by Medicare, but to qualify at first, a physician has to sign a form that indicates that death is likely within six months.) And hospice is a service, it's not a place, though sometimes hospice care is offered at a "hospice." Hospice care can also be offered at nursing homes and in our homes.

Hospice and palliative care focuses on comfort and not on cure. And check this out: patients who demand palliative or hospice care, instead of the fall-back "do everything" position, actually appear to live longer. A study of lung cancer patients who received palliative care had higher quality of life, were in a better mood, and lived nearly three months longer than patients who had standard care.[7] The results extended to spouses, too. In the

National Coping with Cancer Study, when cancer patients die without being put on a mechanical ventilator, having chest compressions, or being admitted to intensive care at the end of life, spouses are three times less likely to develop major depression.[8]

I'd suggest having this conversation earlier than you want to with spouses and physicians. Unfortunately, one woman I interviewed, Peggy Langdon, lost her chance to have the last months with her husband that she wanted. Her husband's treatment team continued to offer new chemotherapy and radiation options even when he was dying. "It was a mistake," she said, and she urged me to communicate that patients near the end of life need greater assertiveness with the medical team.

Some assume that palliative care means only caring about quality of life, and giving up. But palliative care physicians argue that the goal of palliative care is to balance quality with quantity, and that they ask of each intervention: How is this making the patient's life better? Sometimes that means continuing treatment. For example, if chemotherapy reduces the size of painful tumors, we would continue that treatment and we could still say the treatment was palliative.

Unfortunately oncologists are often slow to include palliative care physicians on the treatment team. It can fall to us to ask for this type of treatment. Here's some language I'd suggest using if you find yourself in this position.

"Doctor X, we've talked about it, and it's important to us that if this disease is going to significantly shorten my/his/her life soon, we want palliative care or hospice. We're not giving up, we just want to enjoy whatever time we have left and want to avoid intensive care units. Can you help us make that happen?"

When patients are asked what they want, most of us want to avoid being a burden on our families, don't want to suffer, and want to be conscious—aware of what's happening around us. And yet, too many of us depart like Mr. Jones (a fabricated name), whom I met when I was in training at Harvard. I'd been assigned to the psychiatry consultation-liaison service, which responded to requests from physicians across the Brigham and Women's Hospital to treat patients whose mood appeared to be poor, or who had other psychiatric illnesses.

As it turned out, Mr. Jones, forty-five, had colorectal cancer and was going in and out of consciousness in the intensive care unit. His medical history was thick with attempted and failed treatments, and now he was on heavy pain medications and had just come off of a ventilator, on which he had been dependent for the past two weeks. He was referred when his swearing and sobbing became unbearable for the staff. It was a terrible ending.

Another issue to discuss is how the spouse will feel if the patient dies at home. One young doctor shared with me that his family is very superstitious and relatives would not want to die at home for fear of leaving bad "juju" in the house; as a result, he was inclined to encourage patients to come to the hospital for end-of-life care.

Of course, there are patients who live beyond what is predicted; a large analysis of physicians' estimations showed that roughly one-quarter of the time, physicians underestimate how long a patient will live by four weeks or more.[9] And many patients want to die fighting, if they are going to die. There's nothing wrong with this, as long as it is a conscious decision.

There's also a saying in clinical circles, "People die like they've lived." People who have fought against the world from birth sometimes struggle with the final curtain, and no amount of spousal support can reach them.

## 9-3. Grief is one of the most painful parts of the human experience, but the worst grieving does not last forever.

Just tell people to hang in there, because it does finally get a little better.

—PEGGY LANDGON

No book on couples dealing with cancer would be complete without a section on grief. If you've recently lost your loved one, or are anticipating losing your loved one soon, this is for you.

First, I'm sorry. You're joining a large club of humans. The greatest and hardest experience of our lives is loving someone and losing them. In 1967 the psychologists Thomas Holmes and Richard Rahe created a thermometer of stress with 100 being the absolute worst and 0 meaning no stress at all—and they learned that the number one stressor, at 100, was the death of a spouse.[10] Death was followed distantly by divorce, which they coded at 73.

Let's start with the big picture. Right now, if you are recently bereaved, it probably feels like the world's movie screen is blotted out entirely by your loss. You likely find it difficult to sleep and eat and remember to take your own medications, if you have any, let alone pay the bills or do the laundry.

I promise. Over time, your movie screen will eventually begin to show glimmers of other things again.

The experience of moving ahead through life after the loss of a spouse can feel a little like pulling out of a very tight parallel parking space. You will go a little forward, and then a little backward. And eventually, you'll pull out. But when you go forward a little you'll say, "Wow, I'm getting better!" and then when you go backward, you might say, "I'll never get better." In truth, I don't think we ever fully "get over" a profound loss. It's more like it gets integrated into our lives—we learn to live with it without the burn eclipsing all of our thinking.

It is normal to see and feel the person nearby, to hear their voice, to see them in a crowd, and to talk to them. It's normal to smell them and expect their footsteps down the hallway or hear the way their keys jingled. It's also normal to feel nothing. To feel absolutely numb.

Some writers, like the popular writer Elisabeth Kübler-Ross, suggested that there are common stages of grief such as denial, anger, or bargaining, but this has not been borne out in research. Instead, it looks like we all grieve a little differently. There are two tasks that seem important during the process, however: attaching and separating. We must spend some time attaching to our memories, and some time separating from them. We have to do both.

When my mother died, my father, her mate for more than forty years, was devastated. I still remember the silver wail of his voice at five A.M. the morning after she died. It emanated out of their bedroom as he cried, knowing she would never be there again. For him, the detaching was seeing someone in his life outside of home every day. He tried to have at least one meal away from the house with neighbors, friends, or other family. He walked every day, and slowly, his life returned.

Here are some other patterns. People who lose their spouses before age seventy appear to do worse than those who lose their spouses later. People who have unresolved issues with their spouse, say from an affair or other marital problems, also appear to struggle more. People who blame themselves in some way or who watched their spouse suffer a great deal also do less well.

After a death, some spouses wonder why they should keep living. This search for meaning is important and makes a difference in the quality of our lives and our drive. Viktor Frankl, a young doctor who was imprisoned in three different concentration camps including the notorious Auschwitz during World War II, discovered, much to his surprise, that some young strapping men quickly became ill and died in the camps while some old women lived. And he puzzled about this until he began speaking with inmates. He learned that those who had a reason for surviving, something they lived for, often successfully endured the camps, while those who had no such drive perished.

In the shadow of a lover's death, finding this meaning can be daunting. Sometimes the meaning is found simply in remembering that living on is what your spouse would have wanted for you. It can also be found in children, grandchildren, parents, or others who need us. For others, it is an opportunity to try new activities that are helpful to someone else. Volunteering, returning to work, or finding ways to help organizations that battle cancer can also be helpful in this search. Finally, some spouses decide to throw themselves into an activity they've always wanted to try but have never had the time or opportunity to pursue. I've had patients who started hiking, bird-watching, or playing competitive Scrabble. And I've had those who took on more daring new activities and become scuba divers, spelunkers (cave climbers), and pilots.

Sometimes it is helpful to be around others who are also grieving. Hearing one's thoughts come out of someone else's mouth can be validating. It can be part of connecting. This is especially true when it feels like the world is gallivanting on with indifference while we are stuck in one place, alone with our loss.

Incidentally, when Viktor Frankl returned to Vienna after being liberated from the concentration camps, he discovered that his wife and parents had all been killed in the camps. He went on to remarry, earned a pilot's license when he was in his late sixties, and continued teaching at the University of Vienna until he was eighty-five years old. That's a long-winded way of saying that for many, there is life—even rich life—after profound loss.

# A Few Last Words

**Be generous with your partner, no matter which role—patient or caregiver—they occupy.**

He tells everyone in the world how wonderful I am, but me.

—Linda Spence

We in the marriage counseling business are consumed with communication and understanding the different perspectives of men and women (as in thinking the genders come from different planets), and there's no question that it's helpful to understand various perspectives. But as researchers dig more carefully into the challenging world of complex relationships, we're learning that some simple and old ideas are powerful, and here's one of them. Abraham Joshua Heschel, a leading Jewish philosopher and theologian of the twentieth century, put it well: "When I was young, I admired clever people. Now that I am old, I admire kind people." As it turns out, simple kindnesses and generosity with our spouses are a powerful predictor of the quality of our relationships.

Researchers at the University of Virginia analyzed data following over three thousand husbands and wives. They found that generosity—which they defined as small acts of kindness, routine displays of affection and respect, and a willingness to forgive our spouse for their flaws—is strongly related to satisfaction in the marriage. Generosity also seriously diminishes the chances that a couple will split.[1]

When we're ill, it can be enormously difficult to summon the energy to help our partners do everything that needs to be done. But we can offer them significant helpings of verbal encouragement and kindness. John Gottman and his colleagues who created what they called a "love laboratory" at the University of Washington noticed that successful couples seem to express positive things to their partners numerous times every day, even after conflicts.[2] This is partially a reflection of successful couples feeling kindly toward their partners, so we have something of a chicken-and-egg problem here; but there's no doubt that expressing positive observations to your partner can be helpful, even when you don't have the energy to be helpful in other ways.

So even if you can't do anything else, do this: Be kind. Be generous.

# Notes

What are these? Journals like *Cancer* and *Journal of the American Medical Association* are where researchers publish their findings. To publish, an editor typically reads a manuscript from a scientist or group of scientists and then sends the article to "peer reviewers," who typically don't know the names of the authors. They carefully read the article and decide if it's made a strong enough contribution to the field to warrant publication. In many cases, most, actually, the peer reviewers ask for improvements to the article. Whenever you hear a research snippet on the radio or read one in the paper, there's almost always a fuller published article. These are the names and locations of the articles I cited in the book. In a few cases I wrote some extra sentences about issues that didn't fit in the book but that you might find interesting.

# Introduction

1. Hae-Chung Yang and Tammy A. Schuler, "Marital Quality and Survivorship: Slowed Recovery for Breast Cancer Patients in Distressed Relationships," *Cancer* 116, no. 4 (2010): 1009.

# 1. Things to Know Immediately

1. M. Stiefel, A. Shaner, and S. D. Schaefer, "The Edwin Smith Papyrus: The Birth of Analytical Thinking in Medicine and Otolaryngology," *Laryngoscope* 116, no. 2 (2006): 182–88. Notably, many surgical skills died with the decline of Egyptian civilization, only to be revived about 300 B.C.E. when Hippocrates and his students started doing surgery again. Western sources routinely invoke the memory of Hippocrates, a Greek, when Egyptians were actually the first to have these skills.
2. Donald Oken, "What to Tell Cancer Patients: A Study of Medical Attitudes," *Journal of the American Medical Association* 175, no. 13 (1961): 1120–28.
3. Dennis H. Novack et al., "Changes in Physician's Attitudes toward Telling the Cancer Patient," *Journal of the American Medical Association* 241 (1979): 897–900.
4. February 10, 2010, e-mail from Arnold P. Gold Foundation, results of patient satisfaction survey of six hundred patients. Unpublished in scientific literature.
5. K. I. Pollak et al., "Oncologist Communication about Emotion during Visits with Patients with Advanced Cancer," *Journal of Clinical Oncology* 25, no. 36 (2007): 5748–62.
6. S. Jauhar, "House Calls," *New England Journal of Medicine* 351, no. 21 (2004): 2149–51.

7. Mount Sinai Annual Report (1955), p. 23, cited in Kenneth M. Ludmerer, *Time to Heal: American Medical Education from the Turn of the Century to the Era of Managed Care* (Oxford: Oxford University Press, 1999), 108.

8. Centers for Disease Control (2007). National Hospital Discharge Survey. See Summary tables, www.cdc.gov/nchs/nhds.htm.

9. Donald K. Cherry et al., "National Ambulatory Medical Care Survey: 2006 Summary," *National Health Statistics Reports*, no. 3 (August 6, 2008), www.cdc.gov/nchs/data/nhsr/nhsr003.pdf. See table 28 for a list of mean time spent with physicians by specialty.

10. H. T. Tu and G. R. Cohen, "Striking Jump in Consumers Seeking Health Care Information," *Tracking Report*, no. 20 (August 2008): 1–8.

11. M. C. Dolce, "The Internet as a Source of Health Information: Experiences of Cancer Survivors and Caregivers with Healthcare Providers," *Oncology Nursing Forum* 38, no. 3 (2011): 353–59.

12. Andrea Meier et al., "How Cancer Survivors Provide Support on Cancer-Related Internet Mailing Lists," *Journal of Medical Internet Research* 9, no. 2 (2007): e12. In this study, the author sampled 9 percent of all the messages sent on the ten most popular listserves and coded the content. She found that the listserves had very little off-topic discussion and that most posters offered more support than they requested. The most common topic on the listserve, notably, was how to communicate with health-care providers. Technical advice about how to do something was also common.

13. Jani R. Jensen, Dean E. Morbeck, and Charles C. Coddington

III, "Fertility Preservation," *Mayo Clinic Proceedings* 86, no. 1 (2011): 45–49.

14. J. Donnez et al., "Children Born after Auto-Transplantation of Cryopreserved Ovarian Tissue: A Review of Thirteen Live Births," *Annals of Medicine* 43, no. 6 (2011): 437–50.

15. G. P. Quinn et al., "Impact of Physicians' Personal Discomfort and Patient Prognosis on Discussion of Fertility Preservation with Young Cancer Patients," *Patient Education and Counseling* 77, no. 3 (2009): 338–43.

## 2. Navigating Your Relationship through Early Challenges

1. Tiffany Field et al., "Autistic Children's Attentiveness and Responsiveness Improve after Touch Therapy," *Journal of Autism and Development Disorders* 27, no. 3 (1997) 333–38.

2. Benedict Carey, "Evidence that Little Touches Do Mean So Much," *New York Times*, February 23, 2010, p. D5; Tiffany Field et al., "Massage Therapy Reduces Pain in Pregnant Women, Alleviates Prenatal Depression in Both Parents, and Improves Their Relationships," *Journal of Bodywork and Movement Therapies* 12, no. 2 (2007): 146–50.

3. M. W. Kraus, C. Huang, and D. Keltner, "Tactile Communication, Cooperation, and Performance: An Ethological Study of the NBA," *Emotion* 10, no. 5 (2010): 745–49. Now, to be fair, it's not clear which came first: the touch or the success. At the time of the study, two of the more successful teams in the NBA were the Boston Celtics and the LA Lakers, both of whom touched more than any other teams.

4. Maria Pisu et al., "The Out-of-Pocket Cost of Breast Cancer

Survivors: A Review," *Journal of Cancer Survivorship* 4, no. 3 (2010): 202–9.

5. Richard W. Grant et al., "Impact of Concurrent Medication Use on Statin Adherence and Refill Persistence," *Archives of Internal Medicine* 164, no. 21 (2004): 2343–48; John D. Piette, Michele Heisler, and Todd H. Wagner, "Cost-Related Medication Underuse: Do Patients with Chronic Illnesses Tell Their Doctors?" *Archives of Internal Medicine* 164, no. 16 (2004): 1749–55.

6. John D. Piette, Michele Heisler, and Todd H. Wagner, "Cost-Related Medication Underuse among Chronically Ill Adults: The Treatments People Forgo, How Often, and Who Is at Risk," *American Journal of Public Health* 94 (2004): 1782–87.

7. A. Mehnert, "Employment and Work-Related Issues in Cancer Survivors," *Critical Reviews in Oncology/Hematology* 77, no. 2 (2011): 109–30.

8. Pamela N. Schultz et al., "Cancer Survivors: Work-Related Issues," *AAOHN Journal* 50, no. 5 (2002): 220–26.

# 3. Conquering the Medicine and the Medical Team as a Team

1. Zometa, a brand name for zoledronic acid injection, is a drug used to prevent osteoporosis in women. It is also used to treat bone metastases in patients with breast and other cancers.

2. Sharon Rolnick et al., "Patient Characteristics Associated with Medication Adherence," *Clinical Medicine and Research* 9, nos. 3–4 (2011): 158.

3. Sharon Rolnick et al., "Barriers and Facilitators for Medication Adherence," *Clinical Medicine and Research* 9, nos. 3–4 (2011): 157.

4. Atul Gawande, *The Checklist Manifesto: How to Get Things Right* (New York: Metropolitan Books, 2009), 34.

5. John D. Piette, Michele Heisler, and Todd H. Wagner, "Cost-Related Medication Underuse: Do Patients with Chronic Illnesses Tell Their Doctors?" *Archives of Internal Medicine* 164, no. 16 (2004): 1749–55.

## 4. Learn to Deal with the Emotions

1. J. Kiecolt-Glaser et al., "Hostile Marital Interactions, Proinflammatory Cytokine Production, and Wound Healing," *Archives of General Psychiatry* 62, no. 12 (2005): 1377–84.

2. James A. Coan, Hillary S. Schaefer, and Richard J. Davidson, "Lending a Hand: Social Regulation of the Neural Response to Threat," *Psychological Science* 17, no. 12 (2006): 1032–39.

3. L. M. Thorton, B. L. Andersen, and W. P. Blakely, "The Pain, Depression, and Fatigue Symptom Cluster in Advanced Breast Cancer: Covariation with the Hypothalamic-Pituitary-Adrenal Axis and the Sympathetic Nervous System," *Health Psychology* 29, no. 3 (2010): 333–37.

4. Shelby L. Langer, Michael E. Rudd, and Karen L. Syrjala, "Protective Buffering and Emotional Desynchrony among Spousal Caregivers of Cancer Patients," *Health Psychology* 26, no. 5 (2007): 635–43.

5. D. Spiegel and J. Giese-Davis, "Depression and Cancer: Mechanisms and Disease Progression," *Biological Psychiatry* 54, no. 3 (2003): 269–82.

6. N. M. Bishop et al., "Late Effects of Cancer and Hematopoietic Stem-Cell Transplantation on Spouses or Partners Compared with Survivors and Survivor- Matched Controls," *Journal of Clinical Oncology* 25, no. 11 (2007): 1403–11.

7. Martin Seligman et al., "The Alleviation of Learned Helplessness in Dogs," *Journal of Abnormal Psychology* 23: 256–62.

8. Lyn Y. Abramson, Martin E. P. Seligman, and John D. Teasdale, "Learned Helplessness in Humans: Critique and Reformulation," *Journal of Abnormal Psychology* 87, no. 1 (1978): 49–74.

9. Aaron T. Beck et al., *Cognitive Therapy of Depression* (New York: Guilford, 1979).

10. D. S. Hasin et al., "Prevalence, Correlates, Disability, and Comorbidity of DSM-IV Alcohol Abuse and Dependence in the US," *Archives of General Psychiatry* 64, no. 7 (2007): 830–42.

11. Marilyn L. Kwan, PhD, a staff scientist in the Division of Research at Kaiser Permanente, Oakland, California, presented detailed results of this study at the Cancer Therapy and Research Center–American Association for Cancer Research (CTRC-AACR) San Antonio Breast Cancer Symposium held December 9–13, 2009.

12. C. B. Forsyth et al., "Alcohol Stimulates Activation of Snail, Epidermal Growth Factor Receptor Signaling, and Biomarkers of Epithelial-Mesenchymal Transition in Colon and Breast Cancer Cells," *Alcoholism Clinical and Experimental Research* 34, no. 1 (2010): 19–31.

13. William R. Miller, "Are Alcoholism Treatments Effective? The Project MATCH Data: Response," *BMC Public Health* 5 (2005): 76.

14. S. B. Hammer et al., "Environmental Modulation of Alcohol Intake in Hamsters: Effects of Wheel Running and Constant

Light Exposure," *Alcoholism: Clinical and Experimental Research* 34, no. 9 (2010): 1651–58.

15. Kira S. Birditt et al., "Marital Conflict Behaviors and Implications for Divorce over Sixteen Years," *Journal of Marriage and Family* 72, no. 5 (2010): 1188–1204.

16. Ibid.

17. Elaine E. Eaker et al., "Marital Status, Marital Strain and Risk of Coronary Heart Disease or Total Mortality: The Framingham Offspring Study," *Psychosomatic Medicine* 69, no. 6 (2007): 509–13. This is a profoundly important finding. The researchers were very careful to control for the influence of age, blood pressure, body mass, smoking, diabetes, and cholesterol.

18. Ronald F. Levant et al., "Gender Differences in Alexithymia," *Psychology of Men and Masculinity* 10, no. 3 (2009): 190–203.

## 5. Having a Great Relationship during Treatment

1. Cirran Devane et al., "Move More: Physical Activity, the Underrated 'Wonder Drug,'" *Macmillan Cancer Support* (2011): 1–19. This report highlights evidence reviewed as part of Macmillan's more detailed 2011 report, "The Importance of Physical Activity for People Living with and beyond Cancer: A Concise Evidence Review."

2. S. A. Kenfield et al., "Physical Activity and Survival after Prostate Cancer Diagnosis in the Health Professionals Follow-Up Study," *Journal of Clinical Oncology* 29, no. 6 (2011): 726–32.

3. Xiaoli Chen et al., "The Effect of Regular Exercise on Quality of Life among Breast Cancer Survivors," *American Journal of Epidemiology* 170, no. 7 (2009): 854–62.

4. Victor W. Ho et al., "A Low Carbohydrate, High Protein Diet Slows Tumor Growth and Prevents Cancer Initiation," *Cancer Research* 71, no. 13 (2011): 4484–93.

5. Notably, the California Walnut Commission has supported studies that have shown that ingestion of walnuts may reduce breast cancer risk and slow prostate tumor growth. But until studies are conducted by researchers who are not supported by walnut growers, it's hard to know if this research is trustworthy. In any event, it is likely that eating walnuts is not bad for us, and may be helpful. So eat some walnuts.

6. J. A. Akinsete et al., "Consumption of High Omega-3 Fatty Acid Diet on Prostate Tumorigenesis in C31 Tag Mice," *Carcinogenesis* 33 (2012): 140–48.

7. M. E. El-Mesery et al., "Chemopreventive and Renal Protective Effects for Docosahexaenoic Acid: Implications of CRP and Lipid Peroxides," *Cell Division* 4, no. 6 (2009): 6; C. H. MacLean et al., "Effects of Omega-3 Fatty Acids on Cancer," *US Department of Health and Human Services, Agency for Healthcare Research and Quality, Evidence Report/Technology Assessment* no. 113 (2005).

8. One estimate has suggested that 50 percent of patients develop "chemobrain," but the term is imprecise to researchers because cognitive changes can be caused by so many different factors. For the academic types in the crowd, here are a few strong studies: N. Boykoff, M. Moieni, and S. K. Subramanian, "Confronting Chemobrain: An In-Depth Look at Survivors' Reports of Impact on Work, Social Networks, and Health Care Response," *Journal of Cancer Survivorship* 3, no.

4 (2009): 223–32; Karyn Hede, "Chemobrain Is Real but May Need New Name," *Journal of the National Cancer Institute* 100, no. 3 (2008): 162–63, 169; and C. Soussain et al., "CNS Complications of Radiotherapy and Chemotherapy," *Lancet* 374, no. 9701 (2009): 1639–51.

## 6. Work Together to Get What You Need from Outside People

1. J. W. Pennebaker and J. R. Susman, "Disclosure of Traumas and Psychosomatic Processes," *Social Science and Medicine* 26, no. 3 (1988): 327–32.
2. Roger J. Booth, Keith J. Petrie, and James W. Pennebaker, "Changes in Circulating Lymphocyte Numbers following Emotional Disclosure: Evidence of Buffering," *Stress Medicine* 13, no. 1 (1999): 23–29.
3. Karen A. Baikie and Kay Wilhelm, "Emotional and Physical Health Benefits of Expressive Writing," *Advances in Psychiatric Treatment* 11, no. 5 (2005): 338–46.
4. D. Spiegel et al., "Effect of Psychosocial Treatment on Survival of Patients with Metastatic Breast Cancer," *Lancet* 2, no. 8668 (1989): 888–91.
5. Pamela J. Goodwin et al., "The Effect of Group Psychosocial Support on Survival in Metastatic Breast Cancer," *New England Journal of Medicine* 345 (2001): 1767–68.
6. A. D. Farmer et al., "Social Networking Sites: A Novel Portal for Communication," *Postgraduate Medical Journal* 85, no. 1007 (2009): 455–59.
7. Jacqueline L. Bender, Maria-Carolina Jimenez-Marroquin,

and Alejandro R. Jadad, "Seeking Support on Facebook: A Content Analysis of Breast Cancer Groups," *Journal of Medical Internet Research* 13, no. 1 (2011): e16.

8. Wen-Ying Sylvia Chou et al., "Cancer Survivorship in the Age of YouTube and Social Media: A Narrative Analysis," *Journal of Medical Internet Research* 13, no. 1 (2011): e7.

9. L. L. Northouse et al., "Interventions with Family Caregivers of Cancer Patients: Meta-Analysis of Randomized Trials," *California Cancer Journal Clinics* 60 (2010): 317–39.

# 7. Let's Talk about Sex

1. P. A. Ganz et al., "Life after Breast Cancer: Understanding Women's Health-Related Quality of Life and Sexual Functioning," *Journal of Clinical Oncology* 16 (1998): 501–14.

2. J. L. Stanford et al., "Urinary and Sexual Function after Radical Prostatectomy for Clinically Localized Prostate Cancer: The Prostate Cancer Outcomes Study," *Journal of the American Medical Association* 283 (2000): 354–60.

3. R. Messaoudi, "Erectile Dysfunction and Sexual Health after Radical Prostatectomy: Impact of Sexual Motivation," *International Journal of Impotence Research* 23 (2011): 81–86.

4. W. W. Lam et al., "Trajectories of Body Image and Sexuality during the First Year Following Diagnosis of Breast Cancer and Their Relationship to Six-Year Psychosocial Outcomes," *Breast Cancer Research and Treatment* (e-pub ahead of print, accessed December 2011).

5. Ibid.

6. S. Tessler-Lindau, "A Study of Sexuality and Health among

Older Adults in the United States," *New England Journal of Medicine* 357 (2007): 762–74.

7. M. Dorval et al., "Couples Who Get Closer after Breast Cancer: Frequency and Predictors in a Prospective Investigation," *Journal of Clinical Oncology* 20 (2005): 3588–96.

## 9. Navigating Our Relationship at the End of Life

1. K. D. Kochanek et al., "Deaths: Final Data for 2009," *Center for Disease Control and Prevention, National Center for Health Statistics* 60: 3.

2. M. J. Silveira et al., "Advanced Directives and Outcomes of Surrogate Decision Making before Death," *New England Journal of Medicine* 362 (2010): 1211–18.

3. E. Azoulay et al., "Risk of Post-traumatic Stress Symptoms in Family Members of ICU Patients," *American Journal of Respiratory and Critical Care Medicine* 171 (2005): 987–94.

4. J. Mack et al., "Racial Disparities in the Outcomes of Communication on Medical Care Received near Death," *Archives of Internal Medicine* 170 (2010): 1533–40.

5. P. Glare et al., "A Systematic Review of Physicians' Survival Predictions in Terminally Ill Cancer Patients," *British Medical Journal* 327 (2003): 195–98.

6. A. Gawande, "Annals of Medicine: Letting Go," *New Yorker*, August 2, 2010.

7. J. S. Termel et al. "Early Palliative Care for Patients with Metastatic Non-small Cell Lung Cancer," *New England Journal of Medicine* 363 (2010): 733–42.

8. A. A. Wright et al., "Associations between End-of-Life Discus-

sions, Patient Mental Health, Medical Care Near Death, and Caregiver Bereavement Adjustment," *Journal of the American Medical Association* 300 (2008): 1665–73.

9. Glare et al., "A Systemic Review of Physicians' Survival Predictions."

10. T. H. Holmes and R. H. Rahe, "The Social Readjustment Rating Scale," *Journal of Psychosomatic Research* 11 (1967): 213–18.

## A Few Last Words

1. J. Dew et al., "Give and You Shall Receive? Generosity, Sacrifice, and Marital Quality," *National Marriage Project Working Paper* no. 11–1 (2011). Available at http://ssrn.com/abstract=1970016. You'll note that generosity is not the same as what the researchers called "major sacrifice." This same study found that major acts of sacrifice in a marriage, like quitting school to help a spouse get through school, are actually related to lower satisfaction with the marriage.

2. L. Carstensen et al., "Emotional Behavior in Long-Term Marriage," *Psychology and Aging* 10 (1995): 140–49.

# Index

breast reconstruction. *See* mastectomy: and reconstruction

business meeting, having a weekly, 120–21

cancer, ways of thinking about, 102–7

"Cancer 101," 7

care taking, excessive, 194–97

caregivers

doing vs. being, 43–49

not taking mood swings personally, 92–95

CaringBridge, 166–67

chemobrain, dealing proactively with, 140–44

chemotherapy, 36–37

at end of life, 203, 204, 207

children, anticipating and addressing the concerns of one's, 52–56

cognitive impairment. *See* chemobrain

communication

about what you want at the end of life, 202–9

talking things out, 114–17

*See also specific topics*

communication styles, gen-

der-specific, 43, 47, 49, 116.
*See also* caregivers: doing vs. being

complications, coping with, 78–81

cryopreservation, 29, 31

date nights, 120–22

death, 208–12. *See also specific topics*

decision making

making one's own, 18–21

should not be done while waiting for test results, 41–43

dependence, 192–94

being at peace with, 190–92

excessive, 194–97 (*see also* protection)

depression, treating, 100–102

diagnosis, disclosure of

to others (*see* privacy)

to patient, 9, 10

diet, 110–11, 132–40

digestion, 135–36

dying at home, 208

eating. *See* food

egg freezing, 29

# About the Author

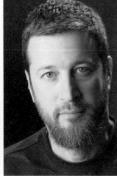

Dan Shapiro, PhD, is an Arnold P. Gold Foundation Professor of Medical Humanism and the chair of the Department of Humanities at Penn State College of Medicine. Dr. Shapiro earned his PhD in clinical psychology at the University of Florida and went on to Harvard Medical School, where he completed an internship and an endowed post-doctoral fellowship in medical crisis counseling. His writings about the patient experience and physician-patient relationships have appeared on or been featured in the *New York Times*, NPR, *Journal of the American Medical Association*, *Salon.com*, *Academic Medicine*, and the *Today Show,* and he is a consultant to the hit television shows *Grey's Anatomy* and *Private Practice*. He also costarred in eight episodes of the *National Geographic* television series *Great American Manhunt* and has appeared on *Dark Matters*, a Discovery Channel science show.

Shapiro has written two other books, both memoirs: *Mom's Marijuana*, about his personal cancer experience (which has been translated into Dutch, Portuguese, Spanish, and Italian), and *Delivering Doctor Amelia*, which focused on his psychological treatment of a physician. He speaks widely to groups of health professionals and patients.

He lives with his wife, Terry, two daughters, a dog, and two cats in Hershey, Pennsylvania. His Web site can be found at www.danshapiro.org.